The Book of Speed
for
Martial Artists

Everything That You've Never Been Taught About
How To Develop Dominating Speed

It's Much More Than Moving Fast

An In-Depth Guide To All Things Speed

David Howell

The Book of Speed for Martial Artists

Copyright © 2017 by David Howell.

All rights reserved. No part of this book may be used or reproduced in any manner whatsoever without written permission except in the case of brief quotations embodied in critical articles or reviews.

For information contact:
CS@TheBookOfSpeed.com
http://www.TheBookOfSpeed.com

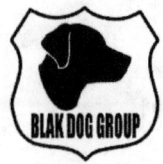

Published by Blak Dog Group LLC

Photography by: Garrett Howell

ISBN-10 : 0692913238
ISBN-13 : 978-0692913239

First Edition: June 2017

10 9 8 7 6 5 4 3 2 1

DISCLAIMER

The content of this book is for informational and entertainment purposes only. It is not a substitute for instruction by qualified martial art, self-defense, and physical fitness instructors. Never engage in martial art, self-defense, or physical fitness training without proper guidance and instruction from a qualified instructor.

The training techniques, exercises, and skills described in this book can be physically demanding and dangerous. You must consult with a medical professional before engaging in any of these activities

Martial arts and self-defense are dangerous, very dynamic, fluid activities that involve countless unpredictable variables, and extreme risk including loss, physical and psychological injury, and death. The author and publisher assume no responsibility or liability for any loss, injury, or death, present or future, that may occur or may be alleged to occur as a result of engaging in these activities or as a result of the application of any of the information in this book. The author and publisher of this book provide no warranty or guarantee, expressed or implied, that the techniques, concepts, or content presented in this book will be effective in any or all martial art or self-defense situations.

The author and publisher of this book are not liable or responsible in any manner whatsoever to any person or entity for any loss, damage, injury, death, or any other adverse consequence of any nature, present or future, that may result from or is alleged to have resulted from studying, practicing, applying or misusing any of the concepts, techniques, or ideas and/or from following any information or instructions contained within this book.

Minors must never engage in martial art, self-defense, or physical fitness training, or any of the training or activities described in this book without responsible and competent adult supervision.

If you choose to engage in any of the activities described in this book or utilize any of the information in this book, you do so at your own risk.

CONTENTS

Introduction.. i
Yeah, introductions are boring. Maybe just speed read it...

Chapter 1
Can You Increase Your Speed?.. 1
Darn right you can. You can have dominating speed.

Chapter 2
Speed Defined... 6
A definition specifically for martial artists.

Chapter 3
Perception to Response.. 12
Doorknobs, diamonds, and guitar players.

Chapter 4
Moving Faster.. 45
Hand speed, foot speed, motor engrams, and silent periods.

Chapter 5
Balance.. 74
The foundation of speed.

Chapter 6
Distance... 100
Be faster without being faster.

Chapter 7
Efficiency... 114
Master this and everything happens faster.

Chapter 8
Strength and Conditioning.. 129
You can't be fast when you're gassed.

Chapter 9
Flexibility.. 140
Get your foot off the brake.

Chapter 10
Mentally Fast.. 147
Get this wrong and nothing else will matter.

Chapter 11
Accuracy and Timing... 159
Missing is speed lost.

Chapter 12
Telegraphing.. 171
Don't give your opponent advance notice.

Chapter 13
Speed and Power.. 179
The speed connection.

Chapter 14
Skills and Training... 195
A box full of speed.

Chapter 15
Speed for Self-Defense... 213
The most important reason to be fast.

Bibliography... 231

This book is dedicated to my two reasons for living:

Garrett and Jenna

INTRODUCTION

Yeah, introductions are boring. Maybe just speed read it...

I STARTED WRITING THIS BOOK WAY BACK IN THE 90s. Unfortunately, my career got in the way, so I set it to the side for many years. It never left my mind though. My goal was always to produce the book I wish had been available to me when I started my study of martial arts.

I've studied the mind, learning ability, and intelligence since the early 80s. That's the same time that I began my study of martial arts. My passion is teaching people how to increase their intelligence, problem-solving ability, and learning speed. I don't say that to impress you, and I'm not implying that my work here is flawless. I say it to give you an indication of my approach to martial arts and the subject of speed.

I'm analytical by nature. For many years, I made my living as a technical problem solver. When I look at something, I automatically analyze it and search for any possible way to make it perform more effectively. The process happens nearly instantly. It's a part of my thinking I cannot and do not want to turn off. So, during my martial art training, I've been constantly focused on the effectiveness of what I was learning and the pursuit of any possible way to make it more effective.

My most trusted instructors have been logic, physics, and body mechanics. I believe that anyone who applies those principals, to the subject of speed, will reach conclusions similar to mine. All I've done here is put those conclusions on paper and added some instruction on how to put them to work. Of course, it will be up to you to adapt the information to your style, goals, and body type, but that's true of everything we do in martial arts.

Please understand that I respect, appreciate, and enjoy traditional martial arts. That may not be apparent at times as you read the pages ahead. When it comes time to fight, you need, above all else, to be effective. Traditional martial arts sometimes fall short. I believe that effectiveness can fit into all martial arts, and speed is a tremendous player in that pursuit.

I'm going to have a lot to say about belief in these pages. Belief is extremely powerful. I was a scrawny, sickly kid. I like to say I was the kid that was getting beaten up by the 90 lb. weaklings. I wasn't considered to be very smart either. I once had a high school teacher tell me loudly, in front of the class, that I was "too stupid to learn." I believed otherwise. I'm not worthy of any pedestals, but I did rack up a very successful tournament record. And, I'm now a member of three prominent high IQ societies. I now teach others how to use their intelligence more effectively. Belief gets 99% of the credit.

You're probably going to grow tired of me talking about conscious thought. Conscious thought is the archenemy of speed, and its ability to slow you down cannot be overemphasized. So, I'm going to denounce it constantly. You're also going to get the idea that I think the solution to *nearly* everything is focused, deliberate training rather than just participation. Well...

Lastly, I want you to know that this book is not a collection of research that I did just so that I could write a book. With the exception of two sections in Chapter 4 and a small reference in Chapter 8, it is entirely a record of my opinions, preferences, and conclusions reached during my personal evaluation and experience. While I learned many things from my instructors, very few of the concepts of speed discussed in this book were among them. In fact, that was my greatest motivation for writing this book.

My intent is for you to find something useful on every page of this book. I certainly hope you find that to be so.

This Is Not A How-To Book

Except for a few training exercises, you will find very few step-by-step instructions in this book. Step-by-step, cookie-cutter instruction is the problem, not the solution. This is a book of knowledge for you to apply to your art, your goals, and your body type. Absorb, apply, experience, and then adapt to you.

*"If I want to teach you, I will **not** answer all of your questions. If I want to cheat you, I will."*

-David Howell

"Absorb what is useful, discard what is not and add what is uniquely your own."

-Bruce Lee

I'm not here to make you "The Drill Master"

I am not a fan of drills. Drills are typically a poor use of your training time. Drills are usually focused exercises that have the goal of improving an isolated aspect of your skillset with the hope that it will translate to actual performance. I believe that is rarely the case.

I'm reminded of the first season of the World's Strongest Man competition in 1977. That season included two of the greatest bodybuilders of all time, Lou Ferrigno and Franco Columbu. It also included a very accomplished weightlifter named Bruce Wilhelm. Wilhelm won the competition in dominating fashion with 63.25 points. Ferrigno finished with 27.5 points and Columbu with 23.25.

All three of these men rose to the top of their sports by lifting weights. The bodybuilders used isolated exercises to focus on development of specific muscles. The weightlifter lifted weights to perfect using his full body to lift large amounts of weight. When it came time to exhibit the ability to lift things and move things with the entire body, the weightlifter's training paid much greater dividends. I have great respect for bodybuilders, but the weightlifter's training simply translated better to performance that required synergetic use of muscular strength.

The bodybuilders' training was analogous to doing drills. The weightlifter's training was analogous to training to do what it is that you intend to do. That's why you won't find drills in this book (for more on why drills are a waste of time, see motor engrams in Chapter 4). You *will* find training exercises that develop effective skills. Look for the words "Train It." These training exercises will have direct correlation to martial arts and your pursuit of dominating speed.

I Want You To Be Able To Get The Newspaper

Students constantly ask me questions like, "If someone attacks me with a knife like this, what should I do?" or "If my opponent throws this kick or that kick, what should I do?" They expect me to show them a scripted defense that they can file away in their mind to have ready to call on if the need should ever arise.

Most students expect their entire training to be a list of when-this-happens-do-this pre-planned, scripted techniques. Some instructors oblige by teaching this way. This makes no sense to me. There are few things as dynamic and ever-changing as sparring, fighting, and self-defense. How can anyone expect to script a response? Worse, how can anyone expect to be the victim of an attack that fits their script? And then, there is the problem of finding a cooperative opponent.

That's why I believe I would be doing you a disservice if I filled the following pages with dozens of still photos of how to do this or that.

Getting The Newspaper

I started responding to those students with a story about a guy who had built himself a robot servant. The robot had twenty buttons on its chest. Each button would send the robot off to perform a specific task. Button one would send the robot to the kitchen to retrieve a drink. Button two would have the robot fetch the guy's slippers. Pressing button three would get the floors vacuumed. Each of the remaining buttons would dispatch the robot to perform a preprogrammed task.

Most people subscribed to newspapers in the 80s when I first started telling this story. Newspapers were printed documents that chronicled the previous day's news. They would be thrown into your front yard in the early hours of the morning. Yes, the 80s were dark and rustic times. Retrieving the newspaper in the morning was often relegated to the family dog because who wants to stagger into the front yard in search of a newspaper first thing in the morning?

This guy wanted his robot to retrieve the newspaper. The only problem was that he hadn't programmed a button for the task of retrieving the newspaper. The robot could walk, it could open doors, it could pick up things, but for all of its futuristic technology, it could not do something as simple as getting the newspaper. It was useless when the situation was beyond its pre-programmed limits.

I would tell the students that I wanted them to "be able to get the darned newspaper, to be able to think for themselves, and adapt." No matter how many "buttons" I help them install in themselves, they would still be useless in all but a few situations, and even those would be doubtful.

Understand

That is one of the most powerful things that you can do, understand. I didn't say understand the instructions you are given. I didn't say understand how to copy what you've been shown. And, I certainly don't mean understand how to memorize scripted and choreographed anything.

No matter what you are learning, understand it as deeply as possible. How, why, and then why again. Do everything you do on purpose, not because it is what you've seen others do, or because it is what you've been told to do. Do it on purpose because you know that it is correct and effective. At the same time, be adaptable, fluid, and ready to respond to any situation.

Knowing is fast, understanding is faster, being adaptable is fastest.

1

Can You Increase Your Speed?

Darn right you can. You can have dominating speed.

I DON'T CARE WHO YOU ARE, OR HOW LONG YOU'VE been a martial artist. You can become faster, probably much faster. In fact, I believe that you can develop dominating speed. And, why wouldn't you want to? Speed is one of the most powerful forces in martial arts. Being faster than your opponent gives you the advantage for offense and defense. Speed can even increase your power for strikes, blocks, takedowns, and nearly every other component of your skillset for any martial art. Speed combined with effective technique is gold for martial artists.

We've got to get past something though, something that you're probably going to get tired of me saying. When martial artists think about speed, they typically are focused on how quickly they can move their hands and feet. They believe that more "hand speed" or "foot speed" will give them the advantage that they seek in the ring and in the street. There is no doubt that hand speed and foot speed can give you a great advantage, but (here it comes) there is much more to speed, dominating speed, than just how quickly you can move your hands and feet. Hand speed and foot speed are extremely important, but don't stop there. They're not nearly enough. Dominating speed is found in the many other places that we're headed to in this book.

Need For Speed

Nearly every instructor tells their students how important speed is. They're right, speed is extremely important. They tell their students they need speed. They tell their students to use speed. They all mean well, but the problem is that they never fully explain speed or how to develop speed. Most of them never go into any detail at all.

It's not because they are incompetent or that they're hiding something. There are a number of reasons why they never actually explain how to develop speed. The first reason is that, to a lot of instructors, a crucial part of learning a martial art is self-discovery through perseverance. In other words, try and fail until you "get it." Some believe that you are either born fast or you're not. There is a little truth in that, but you can still become much faster. So, kick that thought out of your mind right now. Other instructors have just never analyzed speed to the extent that we're going to in this book. They probably even do a lot of what I'm going to suggest, but they've just never taken the time to dissect speed in order to make it easier to comprehend and learn. Then, there are those that teach like they were taught and that's that.

I'm going to do things differently. This book will go far beyond just hand and foot speed. I'm going to tell you every way that I know to increase your speed as it pertains to martial arts. I'm going to tell you why and how. At times, I will go into boring detail. Some of what I cover will be familiar to you, and some of it will be new. I'm going to explain many factors that affect and effect speed for offense as well as defense. Mastering even just one of them can massively increase your speed, and therefore, your effectiveness as a martial artist. If you stop at hand speed or foot speed, you're selling yourself short. But, that's where almost every instructor and student stops. Be one of the few.

So Just How Much Can You Increase Your Speed?

Anybody can improve any of the components of speed described in this book. Don't let anyone convince you otherwise. The degree to which you can, and will, improve will be determined by several factors. Most of them are easily under your control. Others are said to be unchangeable and out of your control, so you should just accept them. Those are the ones that just require a little more effort. All you need to do is identify them and then kick their proverbial butts with knowledge and work.

- **Where you're at now** - The degree to which you have already developed in a particular area determines how much you can improve. If you are already highly skilled in an area, there may be little room remaining for improvement. I didn't say there was no room. I said that there just may be less room.
- **Your body condition** – This means your condition, not your conditioning. Conditioning can always be improved. The effects of aging, accumulated injuries, physical disabilities, etc. can be a little more difficult. Some of those will always be factors and possibly even limitations. Regardless, never let your assessment of your body, or factors out of your control, prevent you from attempting and achieving.
- **Your commitment to training** – You get out what you put in. Simple as that.
- **Your beliefs** – Belief will have a massive impact on your success. It can also doom you to failure. Belief works both ways. Don't let your beliefs control you. Take control of your beliefs by deciding what you believe. Never give in to limiting beliefs. Most often, they're just plain wrong.
- **Understanding** – Do you want to follow step-by-step instructions, or do you want to understand? Understanding will propel you to levels few achieve. Cookie-cutter instructions will just make you one of the crowd.
- **Genetics** – There are some limitations that are carved in stone.

So what? You're not going to let that stop you, are you? Don't stop training until you are certain that you have reached your full genetic potential. Few people ever get there. Then, find ways to augment that level of ability.

It's A Game Of Milliseconds

Watch sprinters and swimmers compete. The winners and losers are typically separated by tiny fractions of a second. The winners are those who mastered the small details that got them to the finish line just that much quicker than their competition.

Martial art speed training is very similar. There are many easy changes you can quickly make that will add tremendous speed to your performance. Then, there are the small details that few will master. Those are the details that will give you a speed advantage over even very accomplished opponents.

To The Doubters

There are many who disagree with my belief that you can become faster. Most of them are fixated on physical speed, which they believe is genetically set. They like to say that you're either born fast or you're not. If physical speed cannot be increased, that means that everyone is as fast as they are ever going to be. If that's so, why do sprinters train? They should just sit on the sofa throwing back junk food 'til race time. They can't possibly learn how to move faster. Right?

Wait! Since we now know that we should give up before we even try to increase our physical speed, maybe we can improve our skills, which might translate to more speed. Nah, that can't possibly be it. After all, you don't tie your shoes any faster now than you did on your first try, do you? You don't deliver basic kicks and punches faster now than you did the day you first learned them either. Right? You don't transition from one stance to another any faster than you did as a white belt. Oh well...

I hope you are laughing. Of course, all of that is nonsense. Thinking that you can't move faster as a martial artist is nonsense as well. Not recognizing that there is speed to be gained in improved skills is nonsense too. Now that you know that you certainly can be faster, much faster, do it. Ignore the doubters.

Belief. A Big Part Of Speed Is In Your Head

I know I'm going to lose a few of you that think speed and power only come from sweat and hard work. That belief crap is a waste of time. Yeah, that's why our Olympic teams take dozens of sports psychologists with them. That's why nearly every elite athlete uses visualization, which bolsters skill and belief. That's why fighters trash talk, which is just another way to affirm their belief, while attempting to reduce their opponent's belief. That's why studies have shown that weightlifters lift more after a hypnotist tells them that they can and why they can lift nearly nothing when the hypnotist tells them that they can't.

I think you will agree that a fighter who has any doubt, has lost before ever entering the ring. Belief alone will never win a fight, but doubt can lose one all by itself. It's still a matter of belief.

Maybe some of you would get along with belief better if I called it confidence or being convinced, or if I told you to rely on your training. They're all the same thing. I'm not asking you to sit in the lotus position chanting affirmations. What I want you to do, is to assume an "I'm fast" mindset. That's it. The trick is to keep that mindset 24/7. Maintain it when you don't see results at first. Keep it when you're training, sparring, or learning a new technique. Do that, and your path to much greater speed will be tremendously easier.

2

Speed Defined
A definition specifically for martial artists.

I KEEP SAYING THAT SPEED FOR MARTIAL ARTISTS IS more than hand speed and foot speed. So, what is it then? To answer that, we need to understand everything that affects and effects speed. Then we need a definition of speed that encompasses all of those factors.

Some say that knowledge is power. Knowing isn't enough. There is even more power in understanding. Deep understanding. Deep understanding is in the details. I'm sure that you would prefer to just get on with it and start training, but stay with me. Invest a little time and maybe endure a little boredom. I promise that the payoff will be worth it.

What A Firetruck Can Teach Us About Speed

Your local fire department has a new firetruck that is incredibly fast. It can reach 90 mph in 6 seconds flat and tops out at 120. It's the fastest firetruck in existence. You call 911 and report that your house is on fire. The firefighters leave the station in their new super truck doing all that it can do. Unfortunately for you, they leave the station five minutes late, go 10 miles out of their way, use up all of the truck's water three blocks before arrival, and they go to the wrong address. When they finally make their way to your home, it has burned to the ground.

The truck moved at record speed the entire way, but were the firefighters fast? No, because their execution was completely ineffective. Their timing was off, they took an extremely inefficient path, they expended their power at the wrong time, and they were not accurate. If a slower firetruck had been deployed at the proper time, had taken a direct route, and had been accurately delivered with full power, it could easily have been more effective than the super truck. Did you get that? The slower truck could actually have gotten the job done earlier. That would make the slower truck the faster of the two.

If the super truck had been deployed at the proper time, had taken a direct route, and had been accurately delivered with full power, it could have been devastatingly effective and extremely fast.

Speed, It's Much More Than Just Moving Fast

The firetruck story reminds us that becoming a fast and effective martial artist requires a lot more than moving quickly.

Speed for martial artists starts with quick, knowledgeable awareness (**Perception**). Then, you need to select what needs to be done (**Response**). To execute that response, you need to be in position (**Distance**) and in control of your body (**Balance**). Your body must move freely (**Flexibility**). You must take the most direct route (**Efficiency**) and move without warning (**Telegraphing**). You've got to be physically capable (**Strength and Conditioning**), and you must be precise (**Accuracy and Timing**). To make all of this happen, you've got to be mentally ready (**Mentally Fast**). You must be effective (**Speed and Power**) and, of course, you must be physically fast (**Moving Faster**).

In that last paragraph, you have a list of nearly all the chapters in this book. They are the skills and components you need to become a truly fast martial artist.

It's About Time

Speed, for martial artists, is about time. From this point forward, when you think about speed, think in terms of time. The time from when you become aware of the need to do something (perception) 'til you get it done (effective completion). For us, that means landing a strike, executing a block, completing a takedown, or whatever else we need to get done. Making it happen in the shortest time possible, that's what being fast is about.

Now we have everything that we need to definitively define speed for martial artists. Our definition begins measuring time at perception, which is the moment that you become aware of something. That something may be internal (in your mind) or external (something your opponent does). The measurement of time stops at the moment that you effectively complete what you chose to do in response to what you have perceived.

> ### The Definition Of Speed For Martial Artists
> *"The time that elapses from perception to effective completion."*

Yeah But...

Some of you may want to correct this definition by starting measurement of elapsed time at initiation of technique, or you may want to add reaction time. Actually, both of these come after perception. Perception of an opening, in the case of offense, or perception of an attack, in the case of defense, are examples of the starting point for measuring speed for a martial artist. Even perception in the form of your own thought or idea to initiate an action starts the clock. The clock always starts once something is perceived.

We Could Argue About When To Start The Clock

We know that speed for martial artists is measured in terms of time. We could argue that the clock should start when a stimulus is presented. In the study of mental chronometry, response time measurements start at this point. After all, that's when the reason to respond comes into existence.

In my definition of speed for martial artists, I start the measurement of time at perception. That's because it doesn't matter when the stimulus is presented. What matters is when you perceive it. Until then, it is out of your control. The time that passes before you perceive the stimulus belongs to your opponent.

Why "Effective" Completion?

We stop measuring time at effective completion because that's what matters. If you are ineffective, you have not completed what you were attempting. Not effectively anyway. The action may end but being ineffective means that it was not completed. The time that matters is the time that leads to effective completion.

It is possible that circumstances may cause you to abandon what you were attempting because you perceived a reason to do so. Time begins elapsing again from the moment you perceived whatever caused you to initiate the new action, even if stopping is the new action. It will end when that action is effectively completed.

What About When To Stop The Clock?

After we perceive something, we must respond. The important thing to remember is that response is not when time measurement stops for us. In terms of speed for martial artists, time stops when we effectively complete our response. That means it not only had to be an effective choice, it had to be executed effectively. A response is not good enough. It must accomplish its intended purpose. Then and only then, does the clock stop. This is a good time to mention that choosing to do nothing is still a response, and it may very well be the most effective response.

So, What's The Problem With Reaction Time?

Reaction time, more accurately simple reaction time (SRT), is a measurement often used in efforts to measure the speed of operations in the brain and nervous system, such as in the field of mental chronometry. SRT is typically defined as the time that passes from presentation of a stimulus to response. Some will end time measurement at the initiation of muscular response.

Simple reaction time tests typically have a planned stimulus and a planned single response, such as pressing a button when a light turns on. This test doesn't account for any cognitive time, for assessment of the stimulus, or for cognitive time for response selection. That makes this measurement useless for the fluid events encountered in martial arts.

Choice reaction time (CRT) is slightly more applicable to our purposes. In CRT tests, there are two or more possible stimuli and two or more possible corresponding responses. This means that the time measurement includes the time expended during the cognitive effort required to evaluate the stimuli and to select a corresponding response. The unpredictability of stimuli in CRT measurement has some relevance to our purposes, but it still falls woefully short.

The point here is that reaction time is an irrelevant time measurement for evaluating your perception, or response speed for martial arts where stimuli and responses are extremely unpredictable. The cognitive time required for both perception and response is what you need to be concerned about. As I will repeat often, those are under your control.

This doesn't mean that SRT type activities (not tests) are not useful for training purposes. They are very effective for developing speed for individual techniques where a single technique is executed in response to a single stimulus. This type of training is focused on motor engram development and conditioning rather than the cognitive processes involved in perception and response. See Chapter 4, Moving Faster.

Your Path Is Clearly Before You

To increase your speed, you must reduce the time needed to perceive and reduce the time required to effectively respond. The components of speed that make that happen comprise the speed formula. Perception, response, moving faster, balance, distance, efficiency, strength and conditioning, flexibility, mental speed, accuracy, timing, skills and strategy, and telegraphing are the vital components of the speed formula. Those are the subjects of the chapters that follow. They are everything that you need to be as fast as you can possibly be.

There are two additional subjects that are vital to effectively using speed as a martial artist: power and self-defense. The speed-power connection is often misunderstood and misrepresented, but it's none the less important. Speed for self-defense can be the difference between life and death.

Time And Time Again

I know that I'm repeating myself, but this needs to be at the forefront of your mind continuously when reading this book and when you are training. Time is speed. Find ways to reduce time in every aspect of your art. Find time reductions in every component of the speed formula. Take time advantages away from your opponent whenever possible. Learn to move faster, but constantly think in terms of time.

3

Perception to Response
Doorknobs, diamonds, and guitar players.

HAVE YOU EVER SEEN A FIGHTER WHO COULD counterpunch so fast that the offensive fighter seemed to never get a punch off? It's a beautiful thing to watch. Each time the offensive fighter attempts a punch, the counterpuncher strikes before the attack even gets out of the gate. The offensive fighter appears to be moving in slow motion and inevitably becomes frustrated when every attempt to strike brings an immediate flurry of counter strikes. The fact that the counterpuncher is the second one to move, but is still the one that scores, is what makes it such a dominating performance.

There is a lot that goes into making that kind of performance happen. Timing, fast movement, efficiency, and skill are all key components, but they're not enough. The two fighters are working at approximately the same distance. In the case of a sanctioned match, they are very nearly the same size and of similar physical condition. They both have substantial training. They've most likely trained in similar styles. So, what's the difference? How does one fighter seem to have advance notice of what's coming?

It is perception and response that make this kind of dominating speed possible. The ability to perceive the slightest indication of an impending strike and to respond with an effective counter instantly, nearly automatically, is what makes the difference. That is extreme speed that is nearly impossible to overcome.

This kind of speed isn't just for countering or defense either. To instantly perceive an opening, your opponent's slight loss of balance, brief loss of concentration, or slightly dropped hand is the way to lightning fast offense as well.

So, Why Don't All Martial Artists Perceive That Fast?

Because they don't even try. That isn't meant to be a disparaging comment. It's just a fact. Most martial artists don't try because they are completely unaware of the concepts involved. They simply don't know what they don't know. I've studied many styles at many schools under many instructors. Most of the instructors were very accomplished. Never once, though, was the subject even mentioned. On the other hand, every student that I've ever taught this to has been successful because there is nothing difficult about it.

There is nothing new about learning to perceive fast. It's been a part of traditional martial arts for centuries. Unfortunately, it has been largely abandoned in recent times. Fast perception can be a product of intense training in virtually any sport. Nearly all elite athletes have very highly developed perception skills. The problem is that they typically develop those skills by default, through countless repetitions during sport specific training, rather than as a deliberate part of their training.

You can develop exceptional perception skills much faster by making perception training a deliberate part of your martial art training. This involves developing an understanding of the concepts and processes involved as well as specific physical training. Once understood, it is easily incorporated into your typical training routine. That means it isn't even going to require any additional training time.

An Ace In The Hole

It is unlikely that you are a professional fighter. That means that you are much less likely to encounter opponents that have already developed the skills that we're going to cover in this chapter. That makes this is an easy ticket to dominating your average opponent.

This chapter is about how to reduce both perception time and response time as they directly relate to martial arts. The remainder of this book is primarily concerned with the effective completion portion of the speed formula for martial artists.

Section 1
Let's Understand What We're Working On

The processes that occur in your brain and nervous system when you perceive and respond are extremely complicated. I'm a believer that there is power in understanding. The deeper and more thoroughly you understand something, the more power you have to control and use it to your advantage. So, I would love to dive into a very technical explanation of the cognitive and neurologic processes involved here. In this case, though, I think that it will serve us better to simplify as much as possible and focus on working knowledge and making it happen, rather than getting lost in the details. Still, there is a lot to consider.

There is good reason for taking this approach. Perception and response primarily happen in the brain. To become faster, we need to increase the completion speed of the cognitive processes involved. Your brain works best, and most efficiently when working with images and concepts. It will handle the details for you. For example, if I ask you to imagine a pink elephant sitting on a Harley on your dining room table, your brain will create the finest details of that image instantly all the way down to the chrome components on the bike and the gleam in the elephant's eyes. Conversely, if I tried to describe that image to you, I could spend days describing every detail. And, you would still just get frustrated and finally give up. Same brain, same image concept, but very different outcomes. It's interesting that when trying to use the brain better, simple works best. It helps too that you already do everything that we're going to cover. We're just going to elicit behaviors that you already know. You're just going to use them differently, to your advantage, and on purpose.

Why Not Reaction Time?

Imagine a simple reaction time test (SRT) (this is also covered in Chapter 1). In front of you, is a light that can illuminate red or green. There is a small button placed where you can comfortably reach it. The test starts with the light glowing red. Your job is to press the button as quickly as possible when the light changes from red to green. The only unknown is when the change from red to green will occur. This is a test that is commonly used in the field of mental chronometry to measure psychomotor speed (the speed of physical movement initiated by conscious mental activity). It measures the time from stimulus (the green light) to response (the press of the button).

Because the stimulus is preplanned, no conscious thought is needed for assessment of the stimulus. In other words, you don't need to think about what is a relevant stimulus, and what isn't. That has been decided for you. The response is preplanned as well, so there is no thought needed for selecting a response. Again, no thinking involved. We're left with a time (speed) measurement of mostly hardwired neurologic pathways.

The Short Story

Reaction time tests only test hardwired neurologic circuitry. Most people will perform very similarly. The potential for improvement is negligible if not zero.

So, why try to improve? Easy, we're not trying to improve reaction time. We're trying to improve perception and response times. Those involve cognitive activities that are very much under our control. That means they can be improved.

It's Complicated

In martial arts, our responses are never as simple as pressing a button. Our movements are typically very complex, involving multiple muscle groups. Even a basic punch is complex enough to require hundreds of repetitions to develop working ability and thousands of repetitions to develop competence. If we put a punch in place of the button press, we begin to measure not only the speed of our nervous system and simple cognitive abilities; we also begin to measure our proficiency in performing the complex series of movements involved.

The Short Story

Now, your response time is heavily dependent on your proficiency with the technique that you are executing. If the technique is new to you, you will be slow because substantial conscious thought will be required. In other words, you will need to think about how to get it done. If you've practiced a few times, you will be faster, just a little thinking required. If you've mastered the punch, you will get it done fast. No conscious thinking necessary.

Big deal. Right? Yeah, it is a big deal because now your response time is affected by something that is under your control and that you can be improved. Not impressed yet? Stay with me it gets better.

Pick One, Any One

Now, let's add in response selection. A punch is not the answer to everything in martial arts. You have many responses (techniques) to choose from. When you perceive a stimulus, you must choose one of the many possible responses in your arsenal. If you haven't trained for this the decision is going to require conscious thought and conscious thought takes time. When it is time to respond there is no time available to ponder about what to do.

You not only need to choose quickly; you must choose wisely. Some techniques are more appropriate for the job. Not to mention that you're better trained at some than others. There are some major decisions to be made. Now, you have a lot of potential for improving your response time.

The Short Story

Now, your speed is dependent on choosing quickly and choosing appropriately. Don't forget that your speed also depends on how well you've trained the technique that you've selected.

So, did you select a response that you can fire off instantly with great speed, or did you choose one that you have to slowly fumble through?

The Final Part Of The Process... Actually, The First

Up until now, we've discussed response and response selection. We've not considered the stimulus. In the simple reaction time test, you had only a single stimulus, and you even knew what it would be ahead of time. In martial arts, the stimuli are extremely varied, fleeting, and unpredictable. Not only do you need to recognize the stimulus quickly, you must understand it so that you can coordinate it with your response selection. Is it a strike, an opening, a fake, etc., etc.? If you are untrained, this is going to require tremendous conscious thought. Perception presents a great opportunity for speed improvement.

The Short Story

This is a biggie. If you've got to consciously think about what's happening, it will be over before you can do anything about it. You can't get much slower than that. To perceive quickly, you must understand, and to be fast, you must understand instantly. That happens in the subconscious mind as a result of effective training.

Well... There Is One More Thing

Back to the simple reaction time test. In that test, the stimulus was a light that changed from red to green. To perceive the color change of the light, you need to see the light. In this case, your eyes are the sensing mechanisms that facilitate perception. You've got to use them effectively, or you are not going to be perceiving or responding.

The Short Story

If your eyes are not aimed where they need to be, anything else you've got going for you is useless. This goes for any of your senses that you are using to perceive.

Putting It All Together

The best-case scenario for maximum speed goes like this:
- Without conscious thought, your sensing organs are where they need to be when they need to be.
- You recognize a stimulus with no conscious thought necessary.
- You select a response with no conscious thought necessary.
- You fire off the response with no conscious thought necessary.

Did you pick up on a theme in that list? Conscious thought is the enemy. You must learn to function without conscious thought. You might be thinking this is impossible. It's not. You already do this routinely throughout your day. We'll explore a few of those times in the following pages.

Why Is Conscious Thought The Problem?

Conscious thought is very slow and requires concentration that narrows your focus. Conscious thought is the thought that you are constantly aware of. Most people, when consciously thinking, think in words. Thinking in words is the slowest form of thought. A minority of people will consciously think in images, which is much faster. Unfortunately, it is still far too slow for martial art purposes.

The next problem with conscious thought is that it consumes your awareness. You may believe you can consciously think about multiple things at once, but you are actually only switching from one to the next and back, albeit rapidly. Any time you are consciously thinking about one thing, other things are neglected. In martial arts, this can mean that while you are pondering about your opponent's hands, you may receive a foot to the gut.

Subconscious Thought Is Where Speed Lives

Subconscious thought is tremendously faster than conscious thought. Subconscious thought happens without you being aware of it, which is interesting considering that it's your mind that is doing the thinking.

There are two types of subconscious thought we need to be concerned with. In this chapter, we are most concerned with decision-making that happens at the subconscious level due to training well enough to achieve subconscious proficiency.

The second kind of subconscious activity is what athletes often refer as "muscle memory." Muscles don't have brains, and they definitely don't have memory. What they are referring to are skills that are so deeply learned that they happen as if the muscles have a mind of their own. This level of performance is due to training that has resulted in the development of motor engrams (covered in detail in Chapter 4).

These subconscious abilities are a requisite for speed and peak athletic performance because our conscious minds simply cannot keep up with the speed of most sports. Subconscious proficiency and motor engrams are so fast that they can create the illusion that we are not even involved in the process. It can be as though we're running on automatic.

Fight Like a Guitar Player

Training to not consciously think frees you to consciously think. Fighting often presents unexpected and unfamiliar situations. Those situations typically require substantial conscious thought because you have no planned solutions stored in your permanent memory. If you are untrained, your conscious mind will already be consumed by basic tasks, such as how to defend yourself. If you have, through training, handed those basic tasks over to your subconscious mind, your conscious mind will be free to handle the unexpected and unfamiliar. In other words, give the guitar playing to your subconscious and let your conscious mind handle the heckler who is trying to interrupt your performance.

So, you should fight like a guitar player. All of your skillset is running in the background (subconsciously) like the guitar playing. Your conscious mind is free and ready to deal with anything unexpected or unfamiliar. Only use your conscious mind when necessary. That's because if you lose focus, you have a much higher probability of getting your head smacked than a guitar player has.

There are some pitfalls to avoid when relying on subconscious thought. Your subconscious mind believes what it has been told, and it acts on that information as if it is gospel. It won't check in with you for updates, and it won't hesitate to act if it is in charge of something, no matter if it is right or wrong. For this reason, you must be careful to only place reliable information in your subconscious mind. Additionally, the conscious mind can easily override and negate the subconscious mind, even when it is working in your favor.

Motor Engrams, The Speed Shortcuts

It can be a struggle to learn a new technique. You're typically uncoordinated, inefficient, and you make multiple errors. You're slow. The more you practice, the better you get. Eventually, the technique is quick enough to be useful. Practice a few thousand times, and you can fire it off reliably and fast. Many thousands more and it executes like it's "second nature." Now, you're darned fast. You've built, or are well on your way to building, a motor engram.

A motor engram is what athletes commonly call "muscle memory." They're memories, but your muscles have nothing to do with them. Motor engrams enable movement that is precise and fast with no conscious cognitive effort necessary. We're going to go into much more detail about motor engrams in Chapter 4. For now, let's just think of motor engrams as preprogrammed weapons and defenses that you can fire off at will. Just pick one, and it will get the job done for you automatically. No thought or intervention needed. This is the absolute peak of physical and mental speed.

Perceiving vs. Sensing

Perception happens in the brain and is facilitated by the mind. Sensing happens in the sensing organs. Perception is the process of becoming aware of information supplied by your senses and assigning meaning (understanding) to that information. If you see your opponent's hand move without understanding what the movement means, you have only become aware of the movement. The movement has no meaning to you, so you cannot effectively respond. You won't know if the movement is a threat, a counterattack opportunity, or a distraction attempt. Analyzation, that includes weighing the action against your stored knowledge, results in understanding that constitutes useful perception.

It is very important to understand the difference. Knowing that perception happens in the mind, tells us that there is plentiful opportunity for improvement because the mind has few limits and is easily trained. There is power in knowing that you need to work on your mind as much as your physical body.

Section 2
Perceive Without Conscious Thought

The first step to increasing perception speed is to perceive without conscious thought. This simply means to become aware of something without analyzing it. Pure awareness without thought is the goal.

This is something that your body already knows how to do. Your body is designed for perception without conscious thought as part of its threat detection system. Threat responses must bypass conscious thought to ensure that they are fast enough to be effective. All we're going to do here is elicit that type of behavior deliberately and in our desired field of view. In section 3 we will put it to work for martial art specific skills.

To understand this better let's look at two scenarios. The first, "Play Ball" describes how we typically perceive visually. The second, "What was that?"

describes a scenario that demonstrates your ability to perceive visually without conscious thought.

Play Ball

Imagine that I am standing directly in front of you about fifteen feet away. You are looking straight at me. Unexpectedly I throw a ball right at you. You will analyze the situation in great detail. You will determine everything from the color of the ball to the type of ball to the trajectory of the ball. You will even analyze my body language to further understand what is happening. Your mind will assess countless details about the ball and the entire scene. Even though this happens very quickly, there is tremendous conscious thought involved. You will even be using substantial conscious thought to determine a proper response based on your analysis. Your response will vary depending on the kind of ball that's coming, my demeanor when I threw it, and all of the other data you perceived.

What Was That?

Contrast that series of events with this scenario. This time I am standing fifteen feet away but I am just outside of your peripheral field of view. Unexpectedly I throw the same ball at you that was thrown in the previous scenario. This time you sense the ball as it enters your peripheral vision mid-flight. Your hand will instantly spring up to block the unknown projectile. Your head will begin to turn away instantly, and you may even move your entire body to avoid being hit. The difference is that you won't have any conscious say in the matter. This will all happen before you are consciously aware of the ball or even why you moved. You will be completely left out of the loop.

There will be no analyzation of the ball, no discerning of reasons for the ball's approach, no planning of a response. Your response will be fully defensive, instantaneous, and the result of permanent memory that was standing at the ready. Respond now, ask questions later.

Perception to Response

Think about that for a moment. Your body was directed by your mind to take action before you were even consciously aware that there was a reason. After it was all over your conscious mind was left trying to catch up and was left asking, "What was that?" Bypassing your conscious mind enabled you to respond tremendously faster than in the first scenario. Your response came first with analysis a distant second. This is as fast as you will ever be.

You may be thinking the what-was-that response is a reflex action. You are correct. As you will learn in Chapter 4, all of our movement is based on reflexes.

The Short Story

If something approaches you in a manner that affords you the opportunity to evaluate and understand it, you will. This is typically in your forward field of view. If something approaches you very unexpectedly, as from your peripheral field of view, your body will perceive it and will do something about it without notifying your conscious mind. That tells us that perception is happening beneath our conscious awareness. To be effective that awareness must be functional at all times. That means it is there for us to put to use whenever and for whatever purpose we choose. All we need to do is train ourselves to access it.

The defensive movements during the what-was-that event were effected by dedicated neural pathways (memories) in the brain. We're not concerned with the response at this point. Response will be discussed later in this chapter. In Chapter 4 you will learn how to create dedicated neural pathways for any movement.

This Isn't New To Martial Arts

Martial art masters are often depicted in art and in movies sitting in the lotus position, serenely meditating while staring at a pebble, or other small object, resting in the palm of their hand. The master is not meditating without purpose. The master is endeavoring to perceive the pebble without conscious thought. The master knows this is the key to maximum perception speed. The master knows also all that is needed is to train the mind to utilize this level of perception.

This may sound a little mystical if it is new to you. It is actually very practical and something that is common to high-level athletics, minus the pebble and the lotus position. If batters tried to use conscious thought, every pitch would land in the catcher's mitt. Stay with me, and it will make perfect sense. I can't overemphasize the implications this can have on your pursuit of speed.

Making It Happen

We know we can easily perceive without conscious thought when a threat approaches in our peripheral field of view. So, all we need to do is move that level of perception to our forward field of view and use it on purpose.

This can be a difficult concept to teach. It has been my experience that this is one of those things that you'll get when you get it. Huh? Okay, it's a little like the old "riding a bike" cliché. You can read an entire book on how to ride a bike, but you're still not going to get it until you get it. That happens by doing. And then, once you've got it, you've got it. That's where we're going here.

The pebble meditation is a tried and true way to start. The concept is very sound, but the students that I've worked with have always grasped the concept quicker when using something that is in motion (see Train It #1 below). It's easier to detach conscious thought from the process when there is less time available to focus on the object.

Over the years, I've seen a few amusing drills that try to take advantage of the what-was-that concept. Some of them have you try to catch a ball tossed toward you in your peripheral field of view. Others use small visual cues in your peripheral field to prompt you to execute a technique. The problem is that you know what's coming and approximately when. Not to mention that these are still in your peripheral field. That area already works.

It is useful, however, to elicit the peripheral what-was-that type response a couple of times to solidify your understanding of the concept in order to more efficiently emulate it in your forward field of view. In other words, getting a "feel" for it may help you more quickly recognize it. It's like taking a couple of practice swings before stepping up to the plate. So, enlist a friend to surprise you a few times with an unexpected, and harmless, object thrown at you in your peripheral field when you least expect it.

Perception without conscious thought is not limited to sight. Touch and hearing, which are vital to you as a martial artist, work very similarly. They too can be trained.

Train It #1
The Single Most Important Training In This Book

This might seem simple, but it encompasses the foundation of increasing perception speed. The speed improvement possibilities here cannot be overstated. This is where you become scary fast.

This is where you begin to develop the perception ability that makes the what-was-that response possible in your forward field of view. This doesn't come naturally for most people. The training is simple but the skill you are going to develop often requires substantial dedication. If you don't get this on your first try, don't be discouraged. If you don't get it on your second, third, fourth, tenth, or twentieth try, keep working. Play until you win. If you do get it on your first try, don't stop there. Complacency has no place in your training. Keep improving.

In this exercise, you are going to train your perception of an incoming punch. I don't believe in scripted or choreographed self-defense or sparring practice, but you need to start with something that is a little predictable in order to grasp the concept. Later, we will introduce unpredictability. You must master this skill before you move on. This is the foundation of all perception and response.

1. Stand facing a training partner.
2. Both of you assume a fighting stance.
3. Establish an effective distance from your opponent. Don't reach out and measure with your arm. To read my rant on this practice, see "Stop Extending Your Arm To Measure Distance" (page 113).
4. Aim your eyes where you would typically aim them during sparring. Don't stare at your partner's fist. This training should replicate sparring or a self-defense scenario as closely as possible.
5. Your partner will throw a trailing hand punch at your head or body. The punch can be a reverse, cross, or straight punch. Determine all of this before you begin.

Signal when you are ready at the beginning of the exercise. From that point forward your partner should punch at random times without warning.

6. Your job is to intercept the punch while taking a short step forward as if engaging your opponent. The idea here is to not only work on perceiving the strike but to simultaneously work on taking advantage of your opponent's forward motion and your forward motion to more quickly advance.
7. When intercepting the punch you should block and evade as you typically would during a sparring or self-defense situation.
8. Let your mind go as blank as possible. Anticipate nothing and think of nothing. Just wait. The only thing that you should have planned is the block that you will execute (later you will not even plan this).
9. Relax as much as possible. Your arms and hands should have only enough tension to hold them in position. Open your hands slightly to help you relax your arms.
10. Do not anticipate the punch. You're training perception, not anticipation.

11. Don't look for telegraphs. Perceive only the fist movement. Later, you can do this same training scenario for telegraphs. That would be a great training progression.
12. As your training partner punches, try to perceive the movement of the fist with no conscious thought. Intercept it with a deflecting block as fast as possible while advancing your position.
13. When the punch comes, let your body do the work while your conscious mind is taking a break.

DO NOT CONSCIOUSLY THINK ABOUT WHAT YOU ARE TRYING TO DO.

14. Intercept the punch as early as possible. Your goal is to perceive the punch earlier and earlier. Again, don't anticipate. You're working on perception, not anticipation.

As you progress, have your partner increase the speed of the attack as you increase the speed of your response. Let your mind go blank. Don't look at the punching hand and don't *try* to move fast. Moving fast will come naturally as a part of the process. Let it happen.

Keep it simple. Have your partner confine the attack to a single technique targeted at a single point. As I said before, we will add variations later. Right now, you are only working on being aware of the attack without conscious thought. Your defensive movements are secondary. Even so, this is a synergistic exercise. You are simultaneously working on timing, distance control, blocking, evasion skills, perception, and response.

You should begin to respond nearly instantaneously. You will find yourself intercepting the punch very near the moment that it begins to move. When this happens, you will begin to realize just how fast you can become. And it gets even better.

When To Move On

Keep this in your daily training routine until your partner is moving at maximum speed, and you are consistently intercepting the punch just as it initiates. Then, move to section three below.

If you have trouble clearing your mind, go somewhere else. In your mind, play with your dog, sit on the beach, or walk through the forest. Wherever, you can go and become fully engrossed. All the while continue training. This can get a little dangerous at first so ensure that your training partner knows what you are doing.

Section 3
Let's Get Specific

This section is a continuation of our goal of eliminating the need for conscious thought for perception. In section two, our goal was to perceive movement, in our forward view, without conscious thought. Perceiving movement alone is not enough to effectively respond. We must perceive the movement and understand its meaning. In this section, we will work to add recognition to our perception ability.

If you know something, you don't need to think about it.

We're now able to perceive motion in front of us without conscious thought. That's great, but we now need to add recognition. That means we are going to perceive specific and complex actions with the speed of peripheral perception. Those actions that we need to perceive are sparring, fight, and self-defense specific, such as specific attacks and offensive opportunities. We must not only perceive them; we must identify and understand them to effectively respond. We need to build a database of what constitutes relevant stimuli. As with everything that we're going to discuss in this book, conscious thought is our enemy.

You Know Doorknobs

It's simple. If you see something that is familiar to you, there's no need for you to think about it. When you encounter a doorknob, do you need to stop and think about what to do with it? Do you need to figure out what the thing is? What it's for? How to use it? No. Do you need to measure your distance to reach it? Do you need to take a couple of practice tries before you make a real attempt? Do you need to change your stance? No. You reach out and turn it while you're texting with your free hand and explaining calculus to the friend who's with you. You know doorknobs. Using a doorknob is automatic.

So, if you walked up to that same door, but in place of the doorknob there was a rat trap, three small levers, and ball of twine, you'd stop, stare, and spend some time pondering. For a short time, instead of making progress, you're going to be in what-the-heck-is-that mode, and your mind is going to be going a mile a second searching everything it knows in an effort to make some kind of sense of the situation. When your brain runs out of options in its memory, it will attempt to understand through intense deductive reasoning (conscious thought). There's no doubt that you're not getting through that door as fast as you usually get through doors. Your texting hand will be paralyzed, and your friend is going to wait for that calculus lesson, and instead, is going to be staring at you while you stand frozen and stammering.

Everything's A Doorknob

The idea here is to make as many things as possible, that you encounter as a martial artist, just another doorknob. Attacks are doorknobs, openings are doorknobs. Nothing requires conscious thought because it's all so familiar to you that understanding is automatic. And, understanding is key to perceiving.

Turning Letters Into Doorknobs

Before we get into how to make this happen, let's pick up some clues by looking at a time when you've done this before. A time when you turned letters into doorknobs. This will help us understand what we're going to do with your training.

In the beginning, it's just data. When data arrives from your senses, it has no meaning. For example, the data received from your eyes is nothing more than a graphic representation of the light striking the back of your eye. It is only when you recognize a pattern that matches the knowledge stored in your memory that you can begin to assign meaning to the pattern. It's like when you learned to recognize letters as a child. To you, the letters placed before you were nothing more than random patterns. It was only through training that you began to recognize them and associate them with sounds. To an untrained person, the letters would go unrecognized.

In the beginning, recognizing the letters required tremendous conscious effort. You had little or no knowledge base to draw upon. The knowledge that you did have was fleeting as it had not yet made its way to your permanent memory. Through practice, you eventually moved the pattern for each letter to your permanent memory. Likewise, your knowledge of sounds associated with them as well as the neurological and physiological responses required to produce the sounds were committed to permanent memory. All of this seems simple now, but it was actually a very complex process.

Now, you perceive letters intuitively with zero conscious thought. It all happens without you even being aware of it. Contrast that with the process when you were four-years-old. You looked, you thought, you struggled, and you thought some more. You were agonizingly slow. Errors were plentiful. Now, the entire process happens instantly. You've reached subconscious proficiency. Subconscious proficiency is the ability to perceive (and later, respond) without conscious thought. It happens automatically as if you are not even involved. That is profound. That is peak efficiency. That is when you are extremely fast. And, that is a place that you can take any skill.

Knowing Without Conscious Thought

To be faster than your competition, you've got to instantly perceive what others don't, or at least perceive faster. Most people who walk across a diamond field littered with raw diamonds will see only rocks. Someone with a "trained eye" will instantly see the diamonds among the worthless rocks. An untrained person watching a basketball game will just see people running around bouncing a ball. The nuances of strategy and skill will go unnoticed. An untrained martial artist will not recognize the subtle signs given by an opponent that can be the difference between a win and a loss. You've got to build your database so that you recognize the diamonds (telegraphs, attacks, openings, vulnerabilities, etc.) instantly.

This Isn't An Easy Process To Teach

That's because it is difficult to separate perception from response. When we perceive something, we respond to it. It all happens in a fraction of a second. So, once you understand perception, and later response, you will typically train them together. Still, I want you to thoroughly understand perception independently of response. That's because most martial art students concentrate on response so much that they neglect the nuances of perception. That means this is an opportunity to exceed the skills of your competition.

Perception training is best accomplished during sparring practice sessions that are as realistic as possible and during actual sparring and self-defense practice. Remember that your goal is to build a database of what needs to be perceived. That happens most efficiently when sparring and fighting. Drills are much too contrived and predictable to train anything beyond the very basics of perception.

Let me be clear.
Perception will improve during sparring and self-defense practice over time by default. That's not good enough. Select times to deliberately focus on perception training during your sparring and self-defense training.

Making It Happen

Well… This one is full of hard work. Experience, lots of it, is the only path to turning sparring and self-defense actions into doorknobs and diamonds. There are some ways to economize your time though. They're based in common sense, so they're not exciting but they're none the less powerful.

- Know what you need to know. Be an intense student of your art or sport. Learn from every source possible. Discard what is useless, retain what is important, and master what is essential.
- Keep the goal of building your perception database at the forefront of your mind constantly. Be proactive about it. Study others as they spar and compete in your chosen art. Dissect and analyze their movements. Learn to see the subtle, but powerful, nuances that others don't.
- Don't waste time training anything that is useless.
- Never just spar. Never just train. Every minute must be spent intensely endeavoring to improve.
- Gear up and do it. Take some hits. The best way to become good at perceiving a head strike is to get hit in the head a few times. Those memories stay with you.
- Repetition. Do it and then do it again. Then do it a lot more.
- Real practice. Spar as realistically as possible, but keep it safe.

Don't forget that perception is about offense as much as defense. Perceiving openings and attack opportunities are just as important as perceiving attacks.

Train It #2
If You're Not Ready For Sparring

If you are not quite ready for sparring, or if you attend a school where there is no sparring, you can use this exercise. This one is easy. Just expand your use of Train It #1 to include an unpredictable variety of attacks. In Train It #1, you were focused on perceiving the movement of the attack. Here in Train It #2, you are focused on identifying the attack. Even though the emphasis is on identification, you can still respond appropriately too. Like I said before, it's difficult to separate perception and response.

1. Select three to five attacks to train.
2. Replace the punch in step 5 of Train It #1 with the three to five attacks that you have chosen.
3. Your partner will execute those attacks in random order at random targets.
4. Your goals and progression should be identical to those in Train It #1.
5. As you build your perception database add more attacks.
6. Make all of this as realistic and unpredictable as possible.

A Final Semi-Rant

To make all of this happen, you've got to train specifically to recognize what it is that you need to perceive to be effective. I'm sure that you are saying to yourself, "What do you think I'm doing when I train?" Well, what *are* you doing? Are you practicing choreographed movements that have no usefulness in reality? Are you constantly working on something new and mastering nothing? Are you sparring so unrealistically that you are deeply training useless habits? Are you failing to even train for fighting or sparring? If you're doing any of these, you are not training; you're participating. Unfortunately, that is how most martial art students "train."

Section 4
Stop Consciously Thinking

Now that you don't need to think, stop thinking. You've eliminated the need for conscious thought. Great. That is if you're not still consciously thinking anyway. When you're planning your attack, watching for an opening, deciding on your next kick, etc., you will fixate on elements of the fight one after another. This will cause hesitation, and, while you're pondering, you will create gaps in your engagement. During those gaps, you are not even in the fight.

Your training is useless if you let your conscious mind get in the way. When you were in school, did you ever study thoroughly for a test, know the material cold, and still choke? Yeah, it's happened to most of us. The problem is that your conscious mind got in the way. You've got to learn to turn your conscious mind off.

Fear, doubt, pain, unfamiliarity, worry, anxiousness, distraction, frustration, and any other disconcerting feeling can kick your conscious mind into overdrive and turn you into a "deer in the headlights" in spite of your training. Conversely, your subconscious mind will relentlessly get the job done, and it will get it done at peak speed, but only if your conscious mind stays out of the way.

Your conscious mind always has the power to override your training. You must keep it under control.

Making It Happen
1. Trust your training. Don't micromanage yourself.
2. Become very comfortable with losing, pain, fear, frustration, and anything else that comes your way. Read "Enjoy Getting Hit" (page 158).

There are two ways to make this happen:
- Decide to. Wow, that's simplistic. It sure is, but only one in a thousand people will do it. They all can, most just won't, or they think that they can't. Decide and then do it.
- Train to the point that you can confidently depend on your training.

Section 5
Response

There are two primary factors involved in fast response: association and execution. Association with what has been perceived in order to select an effective response and execution of that response. The discussions on perception and the Train Its in section three incorporated response selection. That is because it is very difficult to separate the two. When we perceive something, we respond. Even if our response is to do nothing. That leaves little more to be said, so this will be brief.

Response Selection

Your training is intended to build a database of potential responses, not choreographed, scripted moves, but responses that are fluid, adaptable, and effective. The speed of your ability to select an effective response based on what you have perceived is completely dependent on training effective skills and experience. In other words, you've got to train something that will work, and you've got to train it a lot. Experience, experience, experience. You've got to do what you do and do it often.

The only possible shortcut is to train with the intention of improvement. Most students just repeat. They seldom make improvement a deliberate part of their training. They improve, but they do so slowly by default. Make every sparring session count. Proactively, deliberately learn from every success and every failure during every second of your training.

Fewer Is Faster

When there are fewer choices available, selection happens faster. That's why I like to keep it simple. That and the fact that fancy and complicated requires more time to execute. Narrow your response selection to what works. Being fast and effective is always the foremost goal. Clean out the clutter. Any technique that is not fast and effective should be disposed of. There is no need to have it in the way of fast response selection, and you certainly don't need to waste valuable training time on it.

Motor Engrams

Most of what you need to know about increasing the speed of execution of the selected response will be found in Chapter 4 in the section on motor engrams. That is where you will learn about how to fill your database with self-executing responses that require no conscious intervention. This is where your response time gets massively reduced.

Section 6
Use Your Senses Better

Your senses are first in line during perception, so why aren't they first in this chapter? They aren't first only because there is less opportunity to increase your speed through improvement of sense utilization. Notice that I said "less" not "no," so this is still valuable information. Everything you perceive in this world comes through your five senses. For stand-up fighters, sight is the primary sense used to perceive an opponent. Touch is the second most used sense for stand-up fighters, but it is the primary sense used by ground fighters. Hearing would be the least used. Smell and taste round out the five senses. If you are relying on these two senses, you have bigger problems than we can address here.

Each of your senses operate at different speeds. Touch is the fastest of the senses that we use for fighting followed by hearing and then sight. The speed differences between these are hardwired, meaning that no matter how hard you try to change them, the differences will remain.

Improving Utilization Of Your Senses

Your sensing organs are nothing more than devices that your body uses to perceive the world around you. They passively transmit data to your brain where it is processed. There is little room for improvement of your sensing organs as they are, for the most part, hardwired by your physical makeup due to genetics. There is a finite amount of time necessary for sensed information to travel from your sensing organs to your brain. The best way to improve your sensing organs is to keep them healthy through proper diet, medical care, and protection. You can, however, improve your utilization of your sensing organs. These improvements are limited, but they are easy and can be quite effective.

Eyes

The most important sense during stand-up fighting and during much of the stand-up portion of MMA is sight, so where you're looking is of utmost importance. You are not going to perceive what you don't see (by sight anyway).

So, where should you be looking to ensure that you perceive what your opponent is doing? Ask a hundred instructors, and you will get nearly a hundred answers. In terms of perception, the answer is to look at everything and focus on nothing. That answer sounds like I'm trying to channel a little Zen, doesn't it? Not really. This is something that you already routinely do.

What do you look at when you are walking through a crowded room? Do you stare at one particular person or thing? Do you stare at the back of the head of the person walking in front of you? No, you see the area in front of you without narrowly focusing on any one particular thing. In this manner, you can react to all of the movement within the crowd, even into your peripheral field of view. Fixating on a single person or item in the room will focus your consciousness as well. This narrowing of your awareness and vision will leave you vulnerable to any changes or obstacles outside the narrow area that you are fixated on.

Understand that fixating or focusing on something happens in your brain, not your eyes. This means that it is completely under your control. As for your eyes, focusing on a single point refers to physically aiming your eyes at a single point.

Making It Happen

For sparring, select an area to aim at. For standup fighters, this is typically around the chest or neck area. I prefer to not look directly at my opponent by keeping my eyes aimed low and slightly off center. It really depends on your style. You may think you need to look where most of the weapons are going to be coming from. That does seem logical, but don't forget that other parts of the body often telegraph what's coming. That's why many martial artists prefer looking at their opponent's eyes. Don't forget the feet. Even a boxer's feet (far from their weapons) will often foretell what's coming.

The main point here is to not fixate on a point on your opponent. Notice that I said to select "an area," not a point. Aiming your eyes at a point converges your eyes and narrows your mental picture as well. Looking at an area diverges your eyes and broadens your field of view as well as your area of awareness.

Read this sentence. Now read this sentence while being aware of everything to your left and right, taking in your full field of view. If you are like most people, becoming fully aware of everything in your full field of view required some effort. Most people fixate on a very narrow area around that which they are interested in. When fighting, that leaves you vulnerable from many angles.

Stay calm. Fear and adrenalin will narrow your field of view.

Look At Your Opponent's Eyes? Maybe Not.

Looking at your opponent's eyes is one of the most popular approaches to sight utilization. That's because the eyes often telegraph one's intentions. There are some serious problems with this though. The eyes present a very small area that is easy to become fixated on. That small area is also very close, which causes your eyes to converge. Those two factors can severely narrow your field of view. The eyes are also very high, which can delay your perception of kicks, knees, and even lower hand techniques especially when your field of view is already narrowed. If you choose to look at your opponent's eyes, ensure that you keep your field of view as wide as possible.

If you choose to look at your opponent's eyes, remember that your opponent is likely looking at your eyes. It's just something we humans do when someone "looks us in the eye." Be careful to be non-telegraphic with your eyes unless you are doing so to mislead your opponent.

Use Your Peripheral Vision

This is definitely not for everyone. It can be very risky. Early on, I realized that I perceived quicker when approached in my peripheral field of view. I felt as though I was reacting on pure instinct. I was already fairly fast, but when using my peripheral vision, I could counterstrike before my opponent's strike even reached me. I experienced such a substantial increase in speed that, during sparring, I began turning my head away from my opponent to keep him entirely in my peripheral vision. This was successful for me, but I eventually realized that I could learn to perceive the same way while looking straight on at my opponent, so I abandoned this approach. Also, in humans, the peripheral field is slightly out of focus. This means that there is a great chance of misidentifying what is occurring.

Fast Guys (And Gals) Wear Black

I always wear black gear. I believe that it is more difficult to perceive the movement of black gear when compared to brightly colored gear. This is especially true when wearing a black uniform, which provides a black background for your hands. Perceiving a straight-line punch is difficult already. Add in black gloves cast against a black background, and it becomes even more difficult.

Touch

Effectively utilizing your sense of touch when fighting is all about position. In short, you need to be touching your opponent in the right position to sense subtle changes in movement. For stand-up fighters, the hands and arms may be used, but for ground fighters, the entire body comes into play.

Once you have learned proper position for your style, the only effective way to improve your utilization of touch is through experience. When training, become very aware of your physical contact. Exaggerate your awareness so that you, as much as possible, improve your tactile perception of your opponent's movements. This warrants emphasis. You need to consciously focus on your sense of touch so that your awareness and perception of your opponent grows. Because you will be focusing so consciously on this one sense, you will inevitably reduce your awareness of your other senses. For safety, you must ensure that your training partner understands what you are doing or you can easily be injured.

While training, you must use conscious thought in order to deeply learn. Deeply learning moves what you've learned to permanent memory where it can be quickly accessed by your subconscious mind. Only then, should you work to turn off conscious thought.

Making It Happen

Many martial art styles rely heavily on tactile training. Wing Chun, for example, utilizes drills, such as "sticky hands" to improve tactile awareness. Western boxing and Muay Thai heavily rely on the clinch for control of opponents. All grappling arts inherently use full body tactile training in virtually all aspects of their training. Adding any of these styles to your training will greatly improve your use of touch.

Ears

Hearing is faster than sight. Our hearing is something that most martial artists give little thought to in their training. This gives us an opportunity to set ourselves apart from the crowd. In sparring, it will be a rare occasion for hearing to benefit us, but we are working for every advantage possible. If you wear headgear, your choice of gear can be important. Choose headgear that protects your ears but does not impair your hearing. Look for gear that utilizes a hard shell over the ears that is sufficiently vented to allow sound in.

Section 7
Perceptual Blindness Or I Never Saw It Coming

This is a little-known phenomenon that you need to be aware of when pursuing improvement of your perception speed. Perceptual blindness (also known as inattentional blindness) has nothing to do with your eyes. It is a psychological phenomenon in which one fails to see something that is in plain sight. That means right in front of you, big as day. You may believe you see everything that's going on in front of you but the fact is that you don't. And, that can be a huge problem for a martial artist. This is a filtering function of the mind and is something that we do, unknowingly, routinely. As much as you believe you see everything in front of you, the fact is, you do not. Several factors can cause you to be blind to what is right in front of you. With all of the data your mind is confronted with, it is forced to prioritize and ignore what it deems to be irrelevant. There was a famous test conducted by Daniel Simons and Christopher Chabris that perfectly demonstrates the concept of perceptual blindness.

!!! SPOILER ALERT !!!
Head to YouTube right now to take the test yourself. Search "Daniel Simons" or "Christopher Chabris." You will find video titles that mention "selective attention test" or "monkey business illusion." The videos are only about 1½ minutes long. Watch now before reading any further.

In this test, subjects were asked to watch a video of a small group of people, some wearing white and some wearing black, passing basketballs to each other. The people were very close to one another and randomly circling as they passed the balls. The subjects were instructed to count the passes by those wearing the white shirts. Because the action was very random and a bit complicated, counting required intense concentration. During the video, a person wearing a gorilla suit walks through the scene. The gorilla walks slowly right between the people passing the basketball and even stops to look at the camera and beat his chest. At the end of the video, the subjects were asked if they noticed anything unusual. A reported 50% of the subjects never noticed the gorilla. We're talking about a huge, obvious gorilla right in the middle of the action. There are several other changes during the short video as well. Very few of the subjects noticed those either.

There are multiple competing theories that attempt to explain why so many people did not notice the gorilla. There is, however, consensus that this is a psychological phenomenon which means that this is a deficit in perception that is occurring in the mind, which is brought on by intense concentration on one factor in a scene. The lesson for us though is that if we are paying very close attention to something, we are likely to miss other things that are right in front of us. This is why we must be as aware as possible of the entire scene in front of us without narrowing our attention or becoming fixated on any one aspect of that which confronts us.

Making It *NOT* Happen

Narrowing your focus to your opponent's eyes, hands, feet, or anything else will leave you vulnerable to anything that you are not concentrating, or fixated, on. That narrowing of your awareness happens in your mind. If you find that you are consistently vulnerable to a particular kind of attack, it may be useful to reassess where your attention is fixated.

We know that conscious thought is speed's primary enemy, but narrowing your awareness is nearly as bad. This becomes much worse if you become fixated on a small area. We also know that fixation and narrowing of awareness happens in the mind and is a product of the conscious mind and concentration.

As I will say many times in this book, you must learn to turn off conscious thought. Here, I will remind you that you must maintain broad awareness. If you are consciously thinking things through, your awareness will be limited. This is why you must train to the level of subconscious proficiency. Then, relinquish your actions to the training that you've deeply placed into your subconscious mind. This frees your awareness. And of course, avoid fixating on anything.

Then, you need to come to terms with not being able to perceive everything. It doesn't matter how fast you are, how well you've trained, or how wide your field of view and awareness is; you're not going to see everything that's coming. You're human. Deal with it and move on. Getting frustrated will just cause you to make mistakes and perceive even less. Your speed depends on your ability to maintain your composure.

Section 8
A Couple Of Closing Thoughts

The Fallacy Of Choreography And Scripting

This is what most martial art schools rely on for improvement of perception and response especially when it comes to self-defense. Your opponent attacks you. You perceive the attack and execute a response. These sessions are often HIGHLY scripted and choreographed, and executed with very cooperative opponents. Often, even the opponent's assistance is scripted and choreographed. They're also performed in extremely unrealistic stances and scenarios. When the time comes for you to defend yourself, what could possibly go wrong?

Gear up and make your practice as realistic as possible while keeping it safe. **NEVER, EVER** train something to the level of subconscious proficiency that has no possible chance of being effective. I suppose it's OK to learn scripted scenarios for demos and the like, but do not associate any of that with your actual self-defense or sparring training.

Find Your Own Cato Fong

Cato Fong, played by Burt Kwouk, was a character in the comedic Pink Panther movies back in the 60s. Cato was the Chinese man-servant of bumbling French police detective, Inspector Clouseau' played by the late Peter Sellers. One of Cato's jobs was to keep Clouseau' in top fighting form by attacking him when Clouseau' least expected it. Out of the blue, Cato would come crashing through a wall or jumping across the table at a restaurant to attack Clouseau', screaming all the while. Of course in the movies, this was always at the worst possible time and usually led to humiliation for all involved.

Minus the crashing through walls part, and the humiliation, this is an extremely effective training method for training perception and response speed. The advantage is that nothing is scripted. When your training partner walks by and throws a completely unexpected punch aimed at your solar plexus, you get some live fire training. This kind of training is much more valuable for perception and response speed than anything you will do in a martial art class. This makes your abilities a natural part of you. Nothing is faster than that.

Of course, keep it safe. In my home, we go for the solar plexus. We usually use our fingertips so that the victim receives an uncomfortable penalty for failing to block or evade. It's all in fun, but it has very serious speed benefits.

Utilizing The Flinch Response

I hesitate to even mention this, but it wouldn't surprise me if some of you have thought of this yourselves. So, I think I should cover it. Back in the early 90s, I had the idea of utilizing the flinch response to increase perception and response speed. My idea was to startle a student a few times to discover how they typically flinch. Then, I wanted to design self-defense skills tailored to the student's existing flinch response. I thought that building on the flinch that was already an instant response would be a shortcut to faster self-defense.

I abandoned the idea very quickly. I found that most people flinch to a position that is very ineffective for self-defense. Everything from their posture to their center of gravity to their hand position were all ineffective. The next problem was that the flinch had been learned over many years. It was about as deeply seated as a response could be. Altering it was a futile endeavor. I concluded that the students would be better served to work on new, practical responses and work to overcome, rather than attempt to use, their existing flinch response.

4

Moving Faster

Hand speed, foot speed, motor engrams, and silent periods.

TO BE FAST, YOU'VE GOT TO MOVE FAST. THAT'S what every martial artist wants and that is exactly what we are going to work on here. However, you might be shocked to know that I don't consider moving faster to be the most important part of speed improvement. Huh? A book on speed for martial artists and you don't think moving faster is the most important part? That's right. Moving faster is important. I just don't want you to get stuck here.

Moving fast is just one piece of the puzzle. The other pieces are spread through the other chapters of this book, and they are just as important as this one. Some, like balance, are more important because balance provides the foundation for movement. Accuracy and timing are at least equally important because they facilitate effective completion. Don't despair though. You can move faster, and moving faster has major benefits. Moving faster increases your overall speed. It also can increase your striking and blocking power. Moving fast is a great advantage for effecting takedowns. Additionally, moving faster makes you more difficult to hit, which is always a big benefit.

Having lightning fast hands and feet is where the fun is, but they're nothing more than flash if they're not accomplishing something useful. Unfortunately, most martial artists either train ineffective technique, train ineffectively, or both. This is one of those areas where you can set yourself apart from the crowd. The rest of this book is the "road less traveled." That's because most of the information there is seldom taught or even thought about in relation to speed. Even fewer martial artists will put in the work needed to make the most of it. Let's get you moving at maximum speed, and then, let's add skills that will make you even faster.

The Definition Of Speed For Martial Artists
"The time that elapses from perception to effective completion."

Your Body Type

I don't have a lot to say about your body type. It is what it is. Some body types are better suited to the development of fast movement than others. So what? I'm going to tell you just a little about muscle types, but I am not going to list reasons why you may not be able to move fast. When others talk about body type, they are typically referring to your limits. Most people never come close to reaching their full potential anyway, so those limits are probably far off right now. So, I can safely assume that most of you have room to improve. I want you to kick limiting beliefs out of your head and move forward despite what others think they know about you. You need to decide what you believe about you. Ignore everyone else. Just put in the work and reap the benefits.

Ditch The Twitch

Your muscles are made up of muscle fibers that fall into two general categories, slow twitch and fast twitch. Very simply stated, slow twitch muscle fibers perform better in slow and endurance activities, while fast twitch muscle fibers (there are actually two types) are more effective for short bursts and fast movements. Your genetics have already determined the ratio of these fiber types in your muscles.

It is here that we could get into a very lengthy discussion about your muscles and how to train them. I don't think that is useful. There are some who say that you should train according to the makeup of your muscles. They offer tests to determine your ratio of slow and fast twitch muscle fibers, and then, they recommend specific training regimes and drills based on the outcome of those tests. Those training regimens and drills typically have zero application to martial arts.

My approach is much different. We have very specific goals. We are martial artists, and we want to move fast. Doing a bunch of drills that don't apply to martial arts is, in my opinion, a waste of time. If you are going to put in training time, train specifically for your art so that you improve your physical ability and your skillset simultaneously. If you are inclined to use unrelated drills, at least adapt them to some aspect of your art.

Play Your Hand

The bottom line here is that you've been dealt a genetic hand. What are you going to do with it? I suggest that you play it to its fullest potential. Don't let the results of muscle fiber tests color your belief in yourself. We humans tend to gravitate to the negative. Even if you consciously dismiss discouraging information, it can still have powerful effects on you subconsciously. Even positive information can lead to complacency if only at a subconscious level. Subconscious effects are often much more powerful than your conscious thoughts. A winning hand is the one that you win with. It's not always the best hand.

Go For It

Yeah, I'm getting a little repetitive, but I need for you to get this deep into your mind. Just set your sights high and fight for those goals. Bitterly resist any evidence that you have limitations. What's the worst that can happen? You can reach your full potential and still not be as fast as you want to be. But then, there you are at your full potential. Who knows? You might even exceed your genetic potential. Humans are known to do that. DO NOT LIMIT YOURSELF. Go for it and don't look back. Ignore anyone who tells you that you can't be fast.

But, I'm Too Big To Be Fast

Okay, even with all of that pep talk, if you're big, you're probably still thinking that you can't be fast. There isn't much way around it. Bigger things typically do move slower (it's hard to argue with physics). That goes for people as well. Just watch a flyweight bout and then a heavyweight bout to see the difference. That said, heavyweights can still be very fast. A fast heavyweight makes for a dominating fighter.

I'm reminded of a tournament I competed in shortly before earning my black belt. Another student from my school was there competing in his first tournament. We'll call him Bart (not his real name). Bart was around 6' 2" at maybe 220 pounds of nothing but muscle as far as I could tell. He looked tough and thought he was as well. Not in a bad way. He had just trained hard and was confident in his skills and abilities. Genetics had also been very kind to Bart. He was extremely anxious to compete. It was a chance for him to finally be put to the test, a chance to show what he could do.

Bart was up next. His time had come. He was amped up and ready to fight. And then, his opponent was called to the ring. Bart was devastated. At first, he was just shocked, but then shock quickly turned to outrage. His opponent was not what Bart was expecting. He was an unusually large man with a body that was very nearly spherical. He certainly did not look like an athlete nor a worthy opponent. It was insulting to even get into the ring with this guy. Still, Bart did. And as you may be guessing, it did not go well for Bart. The rotund gentleman was not only skilled; he was agile and very fast as well. His kicks, in particular, were very fast and very well executed. He was large, but he had command of his body and had obviously trained well. Bart was soundly defeated. It was no contest. Not only did Bart's opponent beat him, he looked good doing it. Bart left the ring in disbelief.

Moral number one: Never underestimate your opponent.

Moral number two: Just because you don't have Bruce Lee's genetics, does not mean that you can't be fast.

Section 1
Motor Engrams

Where Maximum Movement Speed Lives

As I mentioned in Chapter 3, a motor engram is what athletes commonly call "muscle memory." Muscles don't have brains, and they definitely don't have memory. When athletes use the term "muscle memory," they are referring to skills that can be executed as if the muscles have minds of their own. The skills execute as if the performer is not even involved. They are extremely fast, and they are very precise. They're as fast as you will ever be.

So, What Exactly Is A Motor Engram?

Simply put, motor engrams are memories. They're just in your brain rather than in your muscles. More accurately, a motor engram is a dedicated neural pathway in the brain that activates a motor activity. Motor activity is movement that can be very complex and can involve multiple muscle groups. In other words, a motor engram is a very well developed memory of how to move a particular way, like when executing a punch. Motor engrams enable movement that is precise and fast with no conscious cognitive effort necessary.

A motor engram is your body's way of creating efficiency in movement. When an activity is repeated many times, your nervous system creates neural pathways dedicated to that activity. Those neural pathways are very deeply planted memories. Motor engrams can be very simple or very complicated. Practice your jab enough, and your brain will develop dedicated neural pathways for the execution of that movement. You now have a motor engram that executes your jab. No longer do you need to consciously think about how to make it happen.

Motor engrams are a requisite for peak athletic performance because our conscious minds simply cannot keep up with the speed of most sports. Subconscious proficiency and motor engrams are so fast that they can create the illusion that we are not even involved in the process. It can be as though we're running on automatic. That is extremely fast.

A Motor Engram Master Class

The late Frederic J. Kottke, MD, Ph.D., was an internationally recognized pioneer and researcher in the field of physical medicine and rehabilitation. His study, teaching, and clinical work dealt with helping patients create motor engrams as a part of physical recovery. Dr. Kottke (1980) authored a paper entitled, "From Reflex to Skill: The Training of Coordination." This article is a master class on motor engrams and, as he affirms throughout the paper, it relates directly to our pursuit of speed.

Let's have a look at what Dr. Kottke had to say and then relate it to our goals.

"All motor activity is based on inherent reflexes and on modification of those reflexes by higher centers" (Kottke, 1980, p. 559).

What This Means To Us

This statement explains the title of the article. Dr. Kottke (1980) goes on to explain that as infants, we have only reflexes. Those reflexes happen as hard-wired reactions rather than as the result of memories or thought processes. It is only when our brain (the higher center) begins to modify, regulate, and utilize in sequence those reflexes that we begin to develop coordination, and therefore, skill. All of us are well beyond that stage of development, but this base knowledge is still useful for understanding the development of our skills as martial artists.

"A motor engram is a pathway of interneuronal linkages involving activation of certain neurons and muscles to perform a pattern of motor activity in a specific sequence of speed, strength, and motion, and at the same time inhibition of other neuron pathways so that muscles which should not be participating in this pattern remain quiet" (Kottke, 1980, p. 553).

What This Means To Us

A motor engram is a circuit that specifically fires specific muscles in a specific sequence at specific speed and strength. At the same time that the circuit activates the needed muscles, it also turns off muscles that should not be involved. Those muscles could inhibit movement or otherwise alter the desired movement. This relates directly to our need to relax antagonistic muscles, which will be discussed throughout this book.

"If the practiced activity has been precise, the engram pattern developed will be precise. If the practiced activity has been crude, the pattern of the engram will be crude. If practice has been erratic, the engram will be poor and unreliable" (Kottke, 1980, p. 553).

What This Means To Us

Precise practice is the only way to build a reliable motor engram. Every repetition must be as exact as possible.

"The most important aspect of practice to develop a coordination engram is the building of inhibition so that muscles that should not participate in the pattern are inhibited. Repetition of precise performance is the only way by

which inhibition of undesired activity can be developed" (Kottke, 1980, p. 553).

What This Means To Us

If muscles are fired that should not be involved the movement will be imprecise and/or impeded, which means that it can be slowed, weakened, or otherwise incorrect. This eludes to the need to keep antagonistic muscles relaxed during practice and unneeded muscles uninvolved. Again, precise practice is the only path to success.

"Automatic neuromuscular activity is the highest level of motor activity. It occurs in the extrapyramidal system, not under the direct consciousness of the individual, but as the result of initiation of an engram. When an engram has been developed, it is executed at a speed and complexity which is far faster than can be consciously observed by the performer" (Kottke, 1980, p. 557).

What This Means To Us

This should get your attention big time. A motor engram produces the highest level of muscular performance possible. The performance level is too fast and too complex for your conscious mind to keep up. It happens in a part of the nervous system that isn't under conscious control. This means that motor engrams are ***your only way*** to peak performance, and they are an absolute must for developing dominating speed.

"A perfected engram is voluntarily regulated only to the extent that it is excited to begin, maintained as long as desired, and discontinued at the termination of the desired performance. If there is recognition of an error to be corrected or if it is desired to change a sequence of patterns, that change can be instituted by substituting individual components of the engram which have been established by prior practice rather than by the conscious monitoring of each muscle in the motor act" (Kottke, 1980, p. 557).

What This Means To Us

We can only control a motor engram to the extent of starting it, keeping it going, and stopping it. If we realize that we are making an error, or if we want to change what the engram is doing for us, we can substitute individual parts of the engram (remember, they can be complex patterns). But, we can only substitute parts that are themselves engrams that have been created through practice. We can't change anything by consciously controlling each muscle.

"Set up conditions for training in which the task is consistently and successfully performed. Remember that the patient learns only by repetition of correct performances. Keep the effort low during learning by limiting speed and force so that precision is maintained and errors are not made" (Kottke, 1980, p. 558).

What This Means To Us

Here Dr. Kottke uses the word "patient." Don't let that bother you. Later, he relates all of this to athletic performance as well.

This is all about creating a precise engram. That means that every practice must be precise and correct. That means that we start off slow and easy. Fast, hard practice that is incorrect isn't going to help you succeed. **This is further evidence that the exaggerated movements often taught to beginners is a complete waste of time and effort.** Start off right, just slower and easier. Only practice correct form, even when beginning. Those are the reps that add to the development of a correct and effective engram.

"Practice at a speed and with a force at which each repetition is successful and precise. Increase speed or force only as precision can be maintained. Thousands of repetitions are necessary to develop an engram which can be repeated precisely with speed and increased force" (Kottke, 1980, p. 558).

What This Means To Us

Get it as correct as possible every time. That means slow it down and use less force if that is what it takes to do it precisely. Only ramp up the speed and power when you can do so and still do it right. Once you are doing reps at full speed and power, plan on doing so thousands of times to develop a reliable engram.

"Increase the intensity of practice as performance improves. Speed and skill in performance are improved only by practicing near the peak of performance. Repeated practice with speed and precision perfects the engram. Frequent practice at the peak of performance is necessary to maintain an engram" (Kottke, 1980, p. 558).

What This Means To Us

This drives home the point that once you reach peak speed and power, you still need to put in the work to reach your full potential. Then, you must continue to practice at that level to keep the engram that you've developed.

"As a crude estimate I would suggest the following relationships regarding the impact of repetition of an activity on the development of an engram: Tens of repetitions produce testing and awareness of isolated performance by a coordination unit but result in little retention. Hundreds of repetitions begin to create a faint and fragile engram which will fade quickly. Tens of thousands of repetitions form a fair engram in which speed and force can begin to increase. One hundred thousand repetitions result in significantly increased skill. Millions of repetitions are required to perfect an engram" (Kottke, 1980, p. 559).

What This Means To Us

This might be a little depressing at first glance. A whole lot of reps are necessary to perfect an engram. Remember, you are actually building a neural pathway in your brain. That requires time. On the other hand, that one hundred thousand mark can be reached in just five years doing two hundred reps per class at two classes per week. That is entirely doable. Not to mention that you are going to be outperforming most of your competitors long before you reach that goal. Most martial art students put in no more than ten reps per class and nearly zero precise reps. If you are on your way to a professional fighting career, you most likely started very young. You've already developed many engrams in your years of practice, so you have a sizeable head start.

"In competitive athletics, such as the Olympic Games today we see the emergence of younger and younger champions, as athletes are selected at an earlier age and then devote more concentrated time and effort to develop specific skills. We also can increase the peak of performance above the usual maximal level by precise and persistent practice" (Kottke, 1980, p. 559).

What This Means To Us

Here, Dr. Kottke relates all of this to the development of Olympic athletes. He points out that we're seeing younger champions. Simply put, the athletes are doing more repetitions because they are starting concentrated practice at a much younger age. Dr. Kottke (1980) also points out that we can increase our peak performance to a *higher level* than the "usual maximal level" by making our practice precise and by being consistent in our practice (p. 559).

Good News, Bad News

Let's read the last sentence of that last quote one more time, "We also can increase the peak of performance above the usual maximal level by precise and persistent practice" (Kottke, 1980, p. 559). An expert in human physical performance and motor engrams is telling you that you can perform "*ABOVE*" the usual "*MAXIMAL LEVEL*" just by developing motor engrams through "precise and persistent practice" (Kottke, 1980, p. 559). That is a big deal. That means not only your coordination but your speed and power as well.

The only bad news is that there is a lot of work ahead. Let's see if we can find a few shortcuts. By shortcuts, I don't mean skipping over some of the work and repetitions. That has got to happen. Period. By shortcuts, I mean ways to be efficient with your time by exerting no wasted effort so that it happens as quickly as possible.

Making It Happen – For This Section

Limit Techniques – You don't need to make everything an engram. In fact, that isn't even possible. We've learned that building motor engrams requires massive repetitions. There are only so many training hours in a day. Limit your motor engram development efforts to skills and techniques that can be breadwinners. These will be your go-to skills, so choose wisely. If you select skills which you can already execute effectively, you will have a head start. Select only as many as you know that you can train sufficiently and consistently. If you get in two hundred reps three times per week fifty-two weeks per year, you're going to accrue 156,000 reps in five years.

Reps In Your Head – Dr. Kottke didn't mention this, but I believe that you can add to your rep count by doing reps in your head. Science has proven that vividly engaging in physical movement in your imagination fires the same neurons as actual physical movement. To me, that means that these reps will serve to solidify the neural linkages that you are trying to build. That builds motor engrams. Just ensure that your mental work is as precise as your physical work. If you begin to wane mentally or get off track, stop. Regroup and start again later.

Do It Slow And Light. Then Ramp It Up – Only go as fast as you can while still accurate and precise. Precision is more important than speed. You are building a motor engram that will facilitate speed. Precision will build the engram, not speed. Only increase the execution speed of your reps as your skill increases. Be patient. The payoff is worth it.

Don't Train Junk – Like the old computer adage "garbage in, garbage out." Only execute reps exactly how you want them. Precise and accurate is now your mantra. If you are tired, mentally off, or injured, stop. Maybe do reps in your head, but stop the physical work. Only execute that which will contribute to an effective motor engram.

Do It Right From The Beginning – I've never agreed with the idea of teaching exaggerated, ridiculous movements to beginners with the plan of teaching them the right way later. I was lucky that the first style that I studied did this much less than typical. Then, I trained in several other styles. Unfortunately, I found the exaggerated way to be the norm rather than the exception.

If we taught basketball dribbling like we teach martial arts, we would have the students standing pigeon-toed with their hands on their hips. Dribbling would be with a perfectly straight arm and initiated by extending the straight arm directly overhead and then flapping the perfectly straight arm down directly in front with no elbow bend. And of course, they would be required to do this for two years or more before we would begin to show them how to correctly dribble. You know, they need to learn the basic components first. Does anybody else find this absurd? Then why, in the name of all that is intelligent, do we do this to martial art students?

Skip The Exaggerated Beginner Way – Need proof. Dr. Kottke made it clear that starting with exaggerated movement is useless. Sure, you learn perseverance and discipline, but you don't learn effective technique. And, you waste valuable training time that could have contributed to the development of useful motor engrams. The exaggerated teaching model is not just flawed; it is just flat wrong. If you want to learn or teach traditional martial arts, that's great. Just get on with it. Teach and do it right from the beginning. Period.

Dump Useless Drills – Only train effective technique. Do what you intend to do. Enough said.

At The Speed, Power, Distance... Train it like you intend to use it. Of course, you've got to keep it slower and lighter when you are beginning. That is so that you maintain precision. When you've developed skill and can replicate the skill with precision and accuracy, train it at the speed, power, and distance at which you intend to use it. That ensures that the motor engram will be effective and that you maintain it.

Did I Contradict Myself?

At this point, you might be thinking that this engram development stuff sounds a lot like the scripting or choreography that I preach against in the rest of this book. You might even be thinking that this sounds a lot like programming buttons on the robot in the story at the beginning of this book.

Well, it is a bit of a fine line. This isn't scripting because we are not creating a scenario of presumed events. We're training skills to use in any scenario. This isn't choreography for nearly the same reasons. Let's say we are training a straight punch. The engram for that punch can be fired in any circumstance in response to any stimulus. It can be combined with any other skill. Scripting and choreography assume set conditions, a set stimulus, and an opponent that is in a predicted position using predicted movements.

The robot story tells about a robot that executes a *task* when a button is pressed. Motor engrams execute *skills*. Those skills can be combined in infinite combinations. Motor engrams can be altered and overridden by other engrams. The robot in the story could only execute predefined tasks with predetermined outcomes with no way to combine skills.

Section 2
The Pre-Movement Silent Period

There are some in the martial art world that believe that the pre-movement silent period (PSP), also known as premotion silence (PMS), may be the holy grail of quickly creating both power and speed. To the scientific community though, it remains a bit of an enigma.

There are many scientific studies that associate PSP with faster and stronger movement, but its true propose and function remains elusive. I'm going to review some of the most pertinent information from the scientific community and then present my ideas on how you might be able to take advantage of this neurologic phenomenon.

What Is PSP?

Limb movement is the result of nerve impulses that activate your many muscle fibers. When it's time to move hard and fast, you would expect substantial nerve activity. Interestingly, many studies have noticed a brief silencing of nerve activity just before such movements. When it is noted, the movement is typically faster and stronger than when PSP is absent.

Imagine you and a bunch of your friends are attempting to lift a car. You are all moving about and adjusting your position when someone yells "lift." As quickly as you can, you each begin to lift, but the effort is loosely synchronized, and therefore, not very effective. Now imagine that same scenario with one addition. Just before the command to lift someone calls for everyone's attention. The group silences themselves, and then on command, they all exert maximum effort in perfect synchronization. The result is a fast, effective lift.

That's the idea behind PSP. In this case, it is your muscle fibers that are being called to action. Some scientific tests have observed a "silencing" of nerve impulses to the agonist muscles (the ones doing the work) a few milliseconds before a maximal effort. Some believe that this silencing allows the muscle fibers to be called into action as a synchronized group, which results in faster, stronger movement.

It's even more encouraging that this phenomenon occurs when your limbs are under light load (like when chambered) and when maximal effort is exerted (like when power punching). Perfect. Sign me up. Unfortunately, even though PSP has been recognized for a few decades, there is still no consensus about its effects. That doesn't mean you should stop reading though. There is more encouraging information than there is discouraging.

What Does Science Have To Say?

A 1983 study by Conrad, Benecke, and Goehmann entitled, "Premovement Silent Period in Fast Movement Initiation" is the most often cited study on PSP. Ballistic elbow movements were studied for both self-paced and reaction time movements. Right out of the gate we get this statement:

"The results indicate that in ballistic movements there is a positive relation between extent of premovement depression of tonic activity and subsequent phasic innervation. The results suggest that in high speed movements where a maximal number of motor units have to be recruited, those motoneurones which are already tonically active have to be released from tonic activity for optimal synchrony" (Conrad et al., 1983, p. 310).

What That Means To Us

When we need to move fast, with maximum power, we perform better when our muscle fibers are released from action briefly and then called into action in synchronization (as a group).

The study also noted that in subjects that exhibited premotion silence (PMS), *"There was no difference in the PMS for self-paced movements compared to movements started by an acoustic stimulus"* (Conrad et al., 1983, p. 311). It went on to say that PMS was more pronounced during extension than in flexion movements. The good news here is that PMS works just as well if we initiate movement or if we move in reaction to a stimulus. Slightly less encouraging is that PMS appears to work better when we punch (extension) than when we rechamber (flexion) and that not all the subjects exhibited PMS. It was however seen in the majority of subjects.

Keep in mind that PSP is only a few milliseconds long. It is imperceptible even to the one for whom it occurs.

A later study by Mortimer, Eisenberg, and Palmer (1987) gives us more insight. In this study, subjects extended by hitting a *"karate bag"* (p. 552). That's right down our alley. Flexion (return force) was expended into a cushion affixed to the subject's chest. Contradictory to the earlier study, this study found that PMS occurred more often in self-initiated movements (58%) than in reaction time movements (29%). This contradicts earlier studies and may mean that we will have more success in producing PMS when we decide to move than when we move in response to a stimulus. This study did find that PMS was produced more often when movements were at peak acceleration, which is just what we're looking for.

In addition to PMS in the agonist, several earlier studies (all the way back to 1928) noted a silencing of the antagonist muscles as well. This makes perfect sense because tension in those muscles would slow movement. This plays perfectly with the need to relax your antagonistic muscles for faster movement. However, this study actually saw an increase in antagonist activity. But, Mortimer et al. (1987) attributed this to their instructions to hit as hard as possible, which they believe caused the subjects to contract the antagonists when readying themselves. Throughout this book, I'm going to tell you to break the habit of tensing before striking because it will always slow your movement.

Due to many observations, including the fact that some subjects were more capable of producing PMS, Mortimer et al. (1987) concluded that PMS is a learned motor response. They surmise that PMS functions when we need *"instantaneous force"* as *"in competitive sports but infrequent in everyday activities"* (p. 553). This further supports the assumption that PMS is learned, which means that it is available to us.

PMS And The Stretch-Shortening Cycle

Walter (1988) concluded in his study that PMS exists *"for movements in both directions"* (p. 577). This contradicts some prior studies but agrees with several others. If true, it is good news for us because we want to rechamber as quickly as we strike. This study used only subjects who could produce PMS at least 50% of the time, so we're not going to gain any insight into whether or not it is a learned response.

Walter (1988) considers two possible explanations for PMS. The first, as mentioned above, speculates that PMS allows muscle contraction to be synchronized for greater force and acceleration. The second considers a mechanical function. In the mechanical function scenario, PMS allows the limb to move in the opposite direction slightly during the downtime created by PMS. This could happen during flexion of the arm (return to chamber). When the bicep (agonist) is silent, the forearm would move slightly opposite of the intended direction due to the effect of gravity. This would slightly lengthen (stretch) the bicep. This would be followed by the agonist burst that would contract (shorten) the bicep. Keep in mind that this is happening in just a few milliseconds, so the stretching movement is nearly imperceptible. This movement is termed the stretch-shortening cycle (SSC). The SSC movement results in the agonist muscle being lengthened slightly. Positive effects of SSC on mechanical efficiency of muscle contractions have also been noted in several previous studies.

Walter (1988) noted that movements that exhibited PMS were significantly faster than those that did not and that PMS appears to work along with SSC to facilitate ballistic movement. The fastest movements were recorded when both PMS and SSC were detected. The fastest of those were recorded when SSC was the fastest. Unfortunately, we appear to have no control over SSC; although, it appears to occur with nearly every ballistic movement. This means that we can count on SSC being present to coordinate with PMS for faster limb movement.

In earlier studies where PSP was observed, the muscles started in a state of mild isometric contraction (like when being held in chamber). A study by Hummelsheim and Hefter (1991) set out to determine if PSP existed before other conditions, such as a sudden change in tension, changing position rapidly after a small contraction, or before slow movements where the muscular tension was steady. These conditions never produced a single PSP. A study by Heinzel, Ross, and Cleveland (2008) took a similar approach to testing the existence of PSP for fast movements when the muscles were already engaging in voluntary movement. As with many prior studies, elbow movement was employed. Heinzel et al. (2008) tested isometric movement that was increasing as well as decreasing followed by a verbal command to execute fast movement. PSP was observed during extension when the triceps (agonist) were either exerting constantly or decreasing exertion. When the triceps were increasing exertion, PSP did not exist. Heinzel et al. (2008) also observed PSP in the antagonistic muscles. It's encouraging that all of this supports the contention that the best way to produce PSP is from a ready state like being in chamber.

Most important to us was the fact that most of the studies I've mentioned noted faster reaction times when the subject executed fast movements while they were exerting no force. This may mean that we respond faster when we are in chamber, exerting no force. This is also more evidence that you must remain relaxed when in chamber.

So, What's The Bottom Line?

All of these studies ended with a shoulder shrug and a bunch of guessing as to why PSP even exists. They're not even completely sure if PSP causes fast movement or if it is just a side effect. That doesn't mean their observations are useless to us. There is valuable information that we can take away from these studies. Because supporting evidence was observed in multiple studies, I believe that we can reasonably accept the following points:
- PSP occurs more when the agonist is under light isometric load, like when holding in chamber.
- PSP occurs in the agonist muscles and antagonist muscles, like when moving from chamber.

- PSP is learned. Maximal striking and blocking movements should be contributory to producing PSP.
- PSP occurs when moving in both directions, as when striking and rechambering.
- PSP occurs most during maximal efforts, like when executing a power strike, or when striking at maximum speed.
- PSP contributes to faster movement.
- PSP occurs more during self-directed movement than when reacting to a stimulus.
- PSP contributes to greater striking power.

Making It Happen – For This Section

Several of the studies concluded that PSP is learned, but not one of them even speculated about how one goes about learning to create PSP, except to note that the movements were similar to those used in sports.

I believe that PSP can contribute to greater speed and power. I'm also certain that it can be learned. Keep in mind though, that those are my personal conclusions based on my experience and my review of many studies including those referenced above.

It helps that attempting to utilize PSP is a very low-risk venture. That's because the training that I'm going to suggest fits perfectly with your pursuit of speed. It utilizes non-telegraphic movement and good form. This means that you've got nothing to lose.

Train It

This is the training method I used for developing speed and power decades before I ever heard of PSP. It's extremely simple, and I know that it is effective. It also fits perfectly into any speed training regimen.

1. Stand at a heavy bag in a comfortable fighting position.
2. Relax. Excessive tension can negate PSP and tension will slow your movement regardless.

3. Don't move. We know that PSP doesn't occur when your muscles are already moving in your intended direction. Remain still until executing the punch with maximal effort.
4. Execute the strike or kick with only forward movement (extension). This has the added benefit of being non-telegraphic.
5. Explode into the strike or kick as fast and hard as possible. Always ensure that you use proper form. See "Visualization" near the end of this chapter for help making this happen.
6. Rechamber immediately and with no unneeded movement. The punch stops, and it returns just as explosively as it was thrown.
7. Execute at least 25 reps every time you train. For each rep reset, relax, and then, explode into the target with more force and speed than in the previous rep. Visualize every muscle fiber firing in unison with maximum effort.

Don't get the idea that you create PSP by standing still. PSP is only about 10 milliseconds long, and it happens without you being aware of it. Standing still is just to ensure that you are not activating the agonist in a manner that will prevent PSP from occurring. The only way you will know that you are successful is to begin moving faster and with more power, which I believe that you will.

Making PSP Usable

Standing still and executing strikes on a bag isn't very practical. I believe that PSP can be reproduced in a typical fighting scenario if you keep a few things in mind. These suggestions are just plain good form regardless of PSP, so you don't need to do anything out of the ordinary. That doesn't mean it's not going to require substantial conscious effort in the beginning. Start slow, train precisely, and train often.

- **Punching** - Your full body is involved in a power punch. That means there is a lot of movement involved. We know that PSP doesn't happen when the agonist muscle is already active in the direction of our intended strike. That means your arm extension must not happen until the last possible moment. The agonist muscles in your arm should be in a mild state of tension in chamber, just enough to maintain position, throughout as much of the punching motion as possible. That means well after your shoulder begins moving your arm toward your target. Then, and only then, explode into your target with full power and speed.

- **Kicking** - Kicks are more difficult because you should be on your toes and moving constantly. That motion can easily negate PSP. However, a properly executed kick, just like a power punch, will hold chamber until the last moment. This delays your opponent's awareness of just where the kick is going and increases your ability to create PSP. Apply the instructions for punching to your kicking motion.
- **Break bad habits** – It's common for martial artists to begin moving a striking limb forward slowly just before executing the strike. This is very telegraphic and negates the possibility of PSP occurring.

Section 3
More Ways To Move Faster

I've made moving faster a chapter unto itself because it is such an important subject, and I know that it is one that will be of great interest to readers. However, moving faster is not a subject that can be isolated. The chapters on flexibility, strength and conditioning, and being mentally fast address factors that contribute to moving faster. Those include freedom of movement facilitated by flexibility, relaxation of antagonistic muscles, strength and stamina, and belief. To learn all that this book has to offer about moving faster, you must apply those concepts as well.

Break The Slow Habit

Often, I get students to start moving fast. Then, we spar. They throw a couple of fast strikes, and then, they start moving slowly again. I remind them, and they throw a couple more fast strikes. Then, it's right back to moving slowly again. Blocks are worse than strikes. Rechambering is worse than blocks. These people have a slow habit.

It is extremely difficult to get people with the slow habit to move fast consistently. It doesn't come naturally to them. Unless you are moving slow to draw an opening, or otherwise deceive or confuse an opponent, I want you to move fast at all times. Every strike goes out and returns at full speed.

Making It Happen

This requires habit development. You need to replace the slow habit with a fast habit. That means you are going to need to put in time and effort. This isn't going to happen in days. It's going to require weeks and maybe months. Find someone to be your coach. Pick someone who won't let you get away with anything. Have your coach beside you as you spar. Your coach must push you to fire every strike, block, kick, and rechamber with full speed. Your coach needs to be intense and very hard on you. When you slow down, your coach should call you out immediately. Yelling is encouraged. It's for your own good. Persist until moving fast is habit.

This doesn't mean that you should throw four hundred strikes per round. It means that the ones you do throw need to happen with speed and conviction, and rechamber the same way.

Conditioning

To be fast, your body must be well conditioned. This goes for your entire body, not just your muscles. Muscles come to mind first because they are the driving force of moving fast. Connective tissues and joints must be well conditioned as well because they translate muscular action to the skeletal system. Cardiovascular conditioning is equally important unless you can consistently get the job done with one or two moves.

Moving fast consumes tremendous cardiovascular capacity. Sure, there are some people out there who, due to genetics, naturally move fast. They don't need all of this conditioning to get the job done. Wrong. To be an effective martial artist, you need conditioning that exceeds that which fortunate genetics may have provided.

Making It Happen

Shadow work is an excellent full body workout for moving faster. Shadow sparring, shadow boxing, and shadow kicking are all excellent. You are training skills, physical conditioning, and speed simultaneously. The key is to be thinking fast the entire time. Don't spend a moment not trying to move faster and faster. Push yourself constantly. Never just workout unless you have reached all of your goals and are just working at a maintenance level. Pushing yourself doesn't mean pushing unreasonably. This can lead to injury. Work safely but progressively harder. Don't forget to include combinations, fakes, blocks, etc. See Chapter 8 for more.

!!! WARNING !!!

When doing shadow work, be very protective of your joints. Throwing uncontrolled kicks and punches into the air can easily destroy your joints. Never fully extend. For example, when throwing a punch, end the movement with your elbow slightly bent. Always control your movements when they reach the desired extension point.

Weight Training For Faster Movement

Can increased strength help you move faster? Is weight training a good idea? These are questions that commonly come up in discussions about moving faster. To avoid being repetitive (as you've noticed I can be when I want to drive home a point), I've addressed this in Chapter 8.

Excess Weight

Earlier, I made the case that you can be big and still be fast. I stand by that claim, but the fact remains that excess weight will make you slower than you would be without it. It's a matter of strength to weight ratio. Put a 10 lb. weight in a backpack, strap it on and spar for a while. If you are small, take it down to a 5 lb. weight. It won't take long for you to realize how much that small amount of weight will slow you down. If you are carrying excess weight, lose it. Remember, millisecond gains are substantial. They add up. Gain every bit of speed you can everywhere you can. If you do decide to lose weight, do it the healthy way. Eat right and move more, but get it gone.

Stay Loose

Try to throw a punch with every possible muscle tensed. Feel fast? Yeah, right. Tense muscles can't move fast. Train yourself to stay loose at all times so that you have full speed available at all times.

If you need some convincing, watch some slow-motion video of Olympic sprinters. Their jaws flap around like they're about to fall off. That's because sprinters know that tension anywhere in their body will translate to tension elsewhere in their body. Even tension in their jaw. They know that tension is slow. After all, sprinting is about nothing but maximum speed, so they need every edge possible.

Don't get me wrong. I'm not suggesting that you leave your jaw that loose when fighting because you will stand a good chance of getting it broken. But, you can keep every part of the rest of your body that loose until it's time to be tense, like at the moment of impact.

Making It Happen

Practice. There's no shortcut. You're going to practice and train until you develop the habit of staying loose. When you feel yourself tensing, stop. Reset and start again. Repeat until you firmly develop the habit.

Search yourself for tension. It's amazing how many places we hold tension without even being aware that we are. Most of us unknowingly hold muscular tension somewhere out of habit. Mine is in my eyes and brow. Others clinch their teeth or press their tongue against the roof of their mouth. Search out every place that you may be holding tension and work hard to release it. They're habits. Ending a habit is never easy. Awareness, diligence, and determination are the path to ridding yourself of any bad habit.

Try the ritual that I go through before kicking. I've found it to be extremely effective. I lift one foot a few inches off the floor and let that leg go as limp as possible. I then shake it as though I'm trying to shake something off my foot. I keep the leg as limp and loose as possible. I do this over and over with both legs. I look a little silly doing this and I've received a little ribbing about it, but the ribbing stops when I start kicking. This is just as effective for your arms and the remainder of your body. This loosening ritual has two effects. It serves to loosen the muscles as well as setting a mental state of looseness.

The Dark Side Of Relaxed Muscles

Your muscles play a huge part in the protection of your joints. Very loose, relaxed muscles offer little or no protection to your joints. That is why knowing when to tense your muscles (especially on impact) is even more important than knowing when, and how, to relax them. Which muscles to tense and when to tense them is entirely dependent on the technique you are executing and the timing of that technique. Ensure that the muscles around your joints are adequately tensed at any time that they are under stress that may result in injury.

Relax And Then Relax Some More

Relax, dang it! I mean it! Relax. I know, I already said to stay loose. That was referring to your muscles. Now, I mean your mind. Any tension in your mind will show up in your body and will slow you down. The more confident you are in your skillset, the easier it is going to be to stay loose when facing an opponent, so train your skills intensely. Learning to turn off conscious thought is the best way to dispense with mental tension. That is covered in several other chapters.

You're Not In The Movies

Relaxing more can be as easy as breaking the flexing habit. Sure, it looks cool in the movies, but that's where it needs to stay. Guys, in particular, have the habit of flexing every muscle they've got when sparring, especially their upper body. I think it just feels stronger to them. It might help if you're planning on covering up and taking hits. If you're planning on doing any moving though, it's downright debilitating. Do whatever it takes to break the habit now. Enlist the help of a training partner or coach. Habits don't go down easily. Plan to put in the work and don't stop until you win.

Visualization

In my work, I teach people how to use their mind for intelligence, learning fast, problem-solving, etc. I can tell you unequivocally that the greatest power you possess is the ability to visualize. Nowhere in your pursuit of speed will that ability payoff more than when you are learning to move faster. The greats in all athletics use visualization proactively to reach heights that others only dream about. There is a reason that our Olympic teams take along multiple sports psychologists to every competition. Visualization is one of their most effective tools. Put it to work for you.

Making It Happen

Explosive movement is your goal, so there's no better image than exploding into your target. Stand in front of a heavy bag. Let your arm go silent and relaxed. While the arm is silent and relaxed, imagine the arm ready to explode toward its target. You actually don't even need to see an image. The act of imagining (thoughts alone) works just as well. Explosions happen instantaneously and with tremendous speed. That is exactly how you are going to deliver the strike into the bag. Now, deliver the strike as explosively as you can. Maybe it's the fastest strike you've ever thrown. Maybe you're underwhelmed and wondering if you've just been punked. Either one is typical. Regardless, keep at it. It will pay off. Because you are letting your striking limb go silent, you deliver the strike void of telegraphing movements as well. You will become faster and faster. It does work.

You may be thinking that you can't do this when sparring, competing, or in self-defense. You're right. This is use of visualization as a training tool. Use it long enough to develop the skill that you're working on. When it comes time to put these skills into practical use, you will be enlisting a mindset rather than a bunch of individual images.

Move Up A Couple Of Weight Classes

Many unsanctioned open tournaments will allow you to move up a weight class. Typically, larger people move slower than smaller people do just due to their greater mass (especially those untrained in how to use their speed). When I was competing in point tournaments I would often compete in more than one weight class. I would compete in my own and then move up one or two weight classes. This paid off in wins nearly every time primarily because very few people train for speed. Especially heavier competitors.

Be careful though. Every now and then I would encounter a larger competitor who had speed as well. This is when I corrected the old adage, "the bigger they are the harder they fall." More accurately it is, "the bigger they are the harder they **hit**." My knack for not getting hit was all that got me through some of those matches.

The Old Ankle Weight Trick

I used to see this one a lot at open tournaments. 2 ½ pound or 5 pound weights were typically used. The idea is to wear ankle weights for an hour or so before your match. Your legs acclimate to the extra effort needed to move. Right before your match, you're to remove the weights. Suddenly, your legs feel lighter than air. You can snap kicks up with unnatural ease. I have to admit that this trick does make you feel fast. Maybe you are actually faster. I've only tried this once out of curiosity, so I can't say for sure. I'm not a fan of tricks, especially ones that can get you injured. I do not recommend this quick-fix method of increasing your speed. An instant gain in perceived speed like this is a great way to rack up an injury. The ankle weights themselves can pose a hazard after you've worn them long enough to become less aware of them. Don't resort to tricks. Put in the work.

At a tournament in the early 90s, I saw a guy who became so accustomed to walking around with his ankle weights on that he forgot to take them off when his match started. As you might imagine, it didn't go well for him.

5

Balance

The foundation of speed.

Y**OU ARE PROBABLY WONDERING, "WHAT CAN** balance possibly have to do with speed?" Balance doesn't just have something to do with speed; balance is the foundation that speed resides on. The martial arts are about movement. Movement requires body control and body control requires balance. If you are serious about being fast, and I mean fast enough to dominate, then you've got to dedicate yourself to developing outstanding balance and the agility that comes with it.

Think for a moment about the fastest fighter that you've ever seen. Do you remember that fighter being awkward or stumbling about? Do you remember that fighter being unable to attack or defend because of losing control of momentum or body position? Or, do you remember that fighter moving with cat-like agility while dominating and frustrating opponents with attacks and defenses that were executed from all angles with speed, power, and accuracy? Yeah, that's what speed looks like when it resides on a foundation of balance.

The Unsung Hero

Balance may not excite you as much as the thought of lightning fast kicks and punches, but it should. Everything that you do as a martial artist depends on balance. To deliver a technique with speed, you must be where you need to be, and you must be able to move where you need to move at the instant that you need to move there. Hand speed and foot speed are useless without balance. A martial artist with exceptional balance can have a tremendous speed advantage.

And It's Easy

Balance is one of the easiest places to find speed. Here's why: Balance is neglected in martial arts training, so developing beyond your competition is often easy. Of course, balance is a part of everything martial artists do. It is focused, deliberate training of balance that is rare. Balance is easy to improve. Even minimal effort will yield substantial positive results in a relatively short time. Once learned, exceptional balance requires minimal maintenance. It's one of those skills that will stay with you, to some degree, for life.

HOW BALANCE IMPACTS SPEED

Mentally

Throughout this book, I talk about how conscious thought is the enemy of speed. Few things will consume your conscious mind more than being off balance. Being off balance evokes a survival response because we instinctively know that when we are off balance, we are in danger. This is especially true when sparring or fighting because being off balance makes us vulnerable to attack and less able to defend ourselves. We instantly become more focused on righting ourselves than defending. The effort to right ourselves can completely consume our conscious mind. Any time spent consciously thinking about balance is time lost, and time lost is speed lost.

Distance

If you are falling backward when delivering a forward technique, the distance to your target will be increased and the impact will be delayed, and therefore, slower. Not to mention that power will be lost. If your momentum is overcommitted forward when you need to retreat, the distance required for the retreat will be increased, which will slow your retreat. Additionally, time will be consumed when stopping your forward motion in order to initiate the retreat. If your limbs must be extended as ballast to recover your balance, those limbs will be at a useless distance until returned to chamber. Once again, time is lost, and therefore, speed is lost.

Timing

When your timing is off, speed is lost because nothing will happen at the correct time. When you are off balance, proper timing is off because timing requires full control of your position and momentum as well as full awareness of your opponent's position and momentum. This is all more difficult when you are not in control of your balance.

Technique Selection

Your choice of technique is a major speed factor. When you are off balance, your technique choice is limited. That limitation may prevent you from using the fastest technique for the situation.

Accuracy

If a technique does not reach its target, it is, by our speed definition, slow. Accuracy suffers greatly when we are not in control of balance because we are not in control of our position and momentum. Imagine pitching a baseball while standing in a boat rocked by unpredictable waves. Now, try it with someone attacking you at the same time. Yeah, it's like that.

Stamina

Performing martial arts with poor balance skills is very physically demanding due to the extra muscular effort required to constantly fight the effects of over-commitment of motion and improper body position. Being off balance also takes a tremendous mental toll, which can be equally, or even more, taxing on your physical stamina. Losing your balance can cause a burst of adrenalin which can be extremely detrimental to your stamina.

Take It As Far As You Want To

The good news is that, like I said above, balance is very easy to improve. The system that allows you to maintain your balance is an extremely complicated interaction involving your senses, neurological system, and muscles. Paradoxically, it is extremely simple to use and train. The old "it's like riding a bike" cliché serves as a reminder that anyone can train themselves to balance in demanding ways. Riding a bike is not a natural human behavior, but nearly everyone finds it easy after a little practice. The question is how far do you want to go? It is very common to learn to ride a bike, but how about a unicycle? How about a unicycle on a tightrope? Or, a unicycle on a tightrope while juggling? Blindfold anyone...? The human body is fully capable of learning all of these skills. It's just a matter of how skilled you want to become. As for your speed, the more highly trained your balance, the faster, and more powerful, you can become. The best part is that, like that old bicycle cliché, once learned, balance will become a lifelong subconscious asset.

Be One Of The Few

Learning to move your hands and feet fast will put you right there with every other martial artist who has done so. Understanding and mastering balance will give you an undeniable advantage that will set you apart from the crowd. That's right, even the crowd that has worked hard to develop fast hands and feet. Most martial artists know that balance is important, but very few of them make a deliberate, focused effort to develop exceptional balance. You can easily be one of the few.

Static And Dynamic Balance

There are two types of balance: static and dynamic. Both are important to martial artists and vital in your search for speed. Static balance is the ability to balance while stationary. Dynamic balance is the ability to maintain balance while in motion. Dynamic balance facilitates agility. Interestingly, improvement of static balance typically improves dynamic balance as well.

Static balance requires the use of muscular effort to control one's center of gravity for the body to maintain a fixed position. Improvement of static balance is relatively easy and just requires practice, and possibly some muscle development (primarily muscles that you've not used in this manner before). Further improvement is accomplished by increasing the difficulty of the practice sessions. See the "Train It" section below.

Dynamic balance puts your muscles into a battle with inertia and centrifugal forces of your own creation as well as forces exerted against you. Your body is constantly contracting and relaxing muscles in concert with information from your senses to maintain balance.

Command of static balance will allow you to relax more, which is imperative for speed. Exceptional dynamic balance allows you to utilize your new-found speed and keep it under your control any time that you are moving, such as when sparring or in self-defense situations.

A Note About Differing Styles

Every martial art has different balance demands. The balance requirements for the take-downs, throws, and take-down defenses of a grappling art are far different than the balance needs for executing the kicks and punches of striking arts. Even among the various arts within those two categories, the balance demands differ greatly. Compare Goju-ryu to Tae Kwon Do to Wu Shu, or Judo to Greco Roman to Jiu Jitsu. Then, there are the mixed martial artists who must meld together the demands of many styles. As you work to improve your balance, adapt the training exercises and suggestions not only to your specific martial art, but also to your style, ability level, and body.

Learn To Spin First, But Differently

Spinning kicks are a great study in how to approach balance. I love spinning kicks. I know that they are not practical for self-defense, but they can be very effective in competitive sparring. My spinning hook was my breadwinner throughout my tournament days.

Spinning kicks are typically taught by demonstrating the kick and then telling the student to practice the kick until they get it. The student receives some guidance along the way, but that's pretty much it. The students will invariably struggle and often they will land on the floor. Power and accuracy are nonexistent because the students have no idea how to control the force of the kick and still maintain balance. Speed isn't even in the realm of possibilities. If you ask one of these students to just spin (without kicking) they typically wobble and struggle. So, they're trying to throw their leg into the air with power and accuracy, and they can't even spin. Does that make any sense? Learn to spin first and learn to spin properly.

You should have no need for your arms so learn to spin with your hands firmly in chamber, or even behind your back. When you don't need your arms for balance, that means two things: 1. You've developed the command of your balance needed to execute spinning kicks with speed. 2. Your hands and arms can remain chambered where they can be used for strikes or blocks, rather than stretched out to your sides where they are useless. That readiness adds to your speed.

The next key factor is to maintain your balance throughout the spin. You should be able to stop or change direction at any moment during the spin. You should be able to come out of the spin in any direction necessary. You must never be at the mercy of the inertia created by the spin or the kick. This mobility adds greatly to the speed of your attack or retreat. Simply learning to spin while in control of your balance can be a game changer for spinning kicks and your speed.

Making It Happen

This lesson is not intended to teach you a fighting stance, how to kick, or even how to spin. For that reason, the stance used in the photos is very generic and basic. The purpose here is to emphasize the elements that you need to apply to *your* stance and *your* style to effect spins under greater control and with greater speed.

Your goals with this exercise are to learn to:
- Maintain your balance throughout a spin.
- Maintain the ability to stop or change direction at any point during a spin.
- Keep your hands chambered throughout a spin.
- Use no commitment of body momentum during a spin.
- Have no need for your arms, as ballast, during a spin.
- Pass your kicking foot very close to your support leg to reduce centrifugal forces.

Isn't that just a step backward?
In the photos that follow it may look like I'm just taking a step backward. Remember, we're working our way to a 360-degree spin that will end with us facing the same way that we were originally. Your trailing foot will be extended behind you the same way regardless of how far you spin. The point here is that I'm maintaining balance and control throughout the spin.

1. Start with a 180-degree spin.
2. Begin in a shallow stance with your knees slightly bent (Fig. 1). Alternatively, you can use a stance that is applicable to your style but don't use an exaggerated or excessively deep stance. Keep it as practical as possible. Hold your hands in chamber. Line up your heels and distribute your weight evenly. It's best if you are standing with the balls of your feet on a line so that you can easily gauge the accuracy of your spin.

You might be thinking that this looks a lot like one of those useless drills that I disdain because we don't fight with our feet lined up. You should be using a set-up for spinning kicks. It is very common, during the set-up technique, to transition to lined-up feet during initiating of the spinning kick.

3. Begin by turning your shoulders 90 degrees into the spin (Fig. 2). Your shoulders will be perpendicular to the line you are standing on. At the same time, pivot on the balls of your feet so that your heels point rearward. Your weight distribution is still 50/50.
4. Lift your lead leg so that your knee is in kicking chamber position (Fig. 3). Your weight is now 100 percent on your support leg. You should be able to stop in complete control of your balance. Your chamber may be lower or later in the kick. Use the chamber that best suits your style.
5. Extend your kicking foot rearward, heel first. Pass your foot very close to your support leg (Fig. 4) to reduce centrifugal forces.
6. Maintain your balance so that you can stop at any point (Fig. 5 and 6).
7. You should be able to stop with the ball of your foot one inch off the floor (Fig. 7) while in complete control of your balance.
8. Touch the ball of the foot down on the line (Fig. 8).
9. Pivot on the balls of your feet while transitioning to 50/50 weight distribution (Fig. 9). You are now back in a shallow horse-riding-like stance with the foot that was trailing, now as your lead foot.
10. To execute a 360-degree spin, just continue the pivot of your support foot and shoulders an additional 180 degrees. Extend and place your foot down just as in Step 8 ending in your original stance. Keep your center of gravity over your support leg until the moment that you pivot your feet back into the shallow horse-riding-like stance.

The Book of Speed for Martial Artists

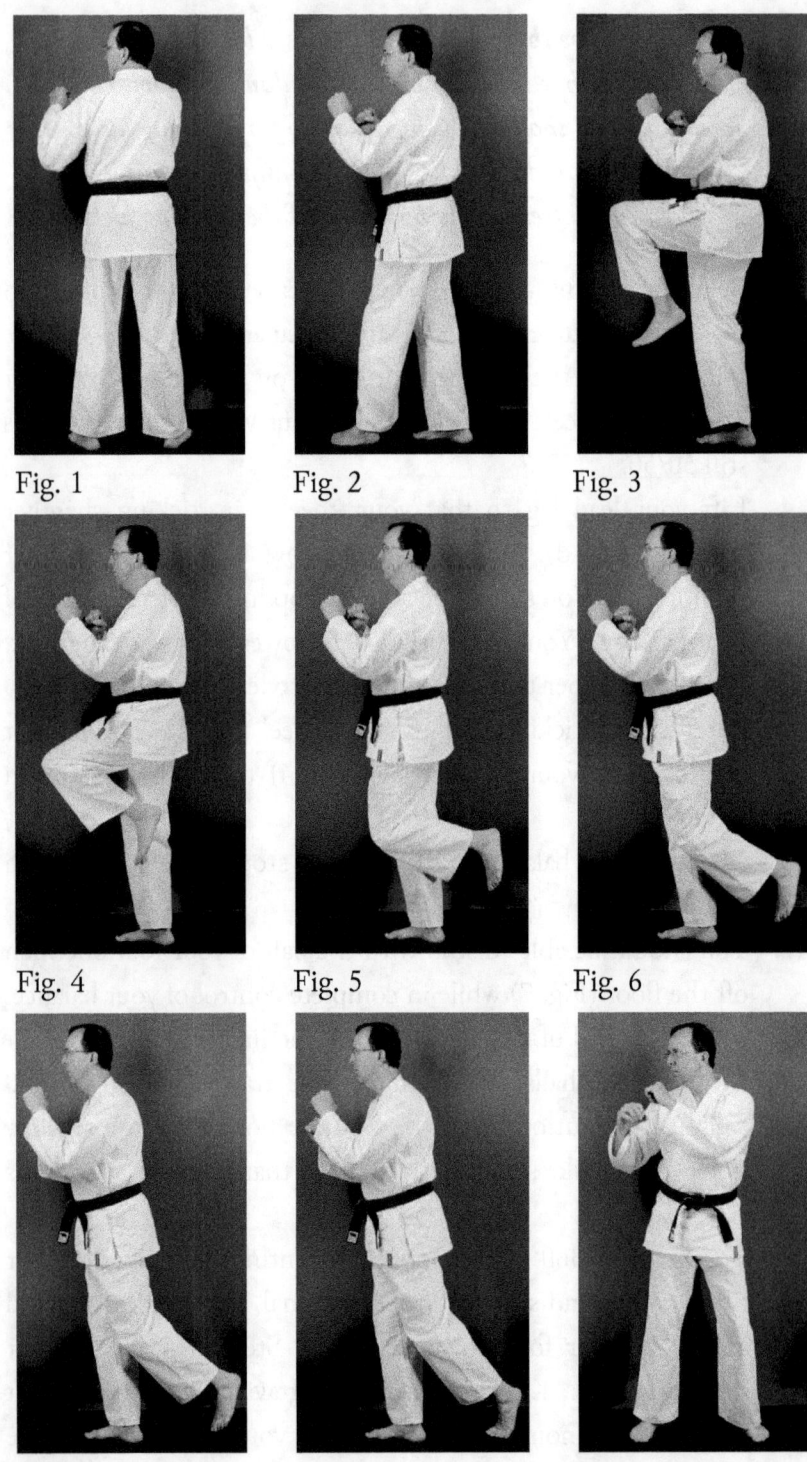

Fig. 1　　　　　Fig. 2　　　　　Fig. 3

Fig. 4　　　　　Fig. 5　　　　　Fig. 6

Fig. 7　　　　　Fig. 8　　　　　Fig. 9

Once you've mastered both the 180 degree and 360-degree spins, begin to add kicks. Only add kicks when you can stop at any point during the spin with complete control of your balance.

Once you add kicks, practice stopping at various points during the kicks. You should be able to stop at any moment with full control of your balance. Practice coming out of the kick in different directions. You should be able to advance straight or at any angle. You can also retreat straight or at any angle. You should have complete mobility during any spinning kick. And, you should have the same control during all of your kicks, spinning or not.

Never allow yourself to be at the mercy of inertia or centrifugal forces.

Reduce Enemy Forces

Often, we are our own worst enemy. We add unnecessary forces, through unnecessary movement and incorrect body positions, that adversely impact our balance. Just reducing those forces through efficient movement can improve your balance dramatically.

Keep it in tight. Don't extend your arms, especially when kicking. Beginners and experienced martial artists alike extend their arms when kicking. For crying out loud, why? Work hard to break this habit. Extending your arms may, at times, assist your balance, but it also adds inertial and centrifugal forces that are far from your center of gravity. These forces require more effort and time to control. Those extended arms also must be rechambered to be useful for striking and defending, which consumes valuable time, further reducing your speed.

If you've ever watched a figure skater spin, you will see that the tighter they pull their arms to their torso, the faster they spin. To slow the spin, they simply extend their arms. You'll also notice that they extend both arms equally. If they were to extend one arm, without altering their body position to compensate, they would be forced into a fall or at least a struggle to regain their balance.

Making It Happen

Every time you kick, keep your hands and arms exactly where you would keep them in your fighting position. When practicing and when sparring, keep them where they belong. The only time they should be anywhere else is when you are using them to execute a useful technique.

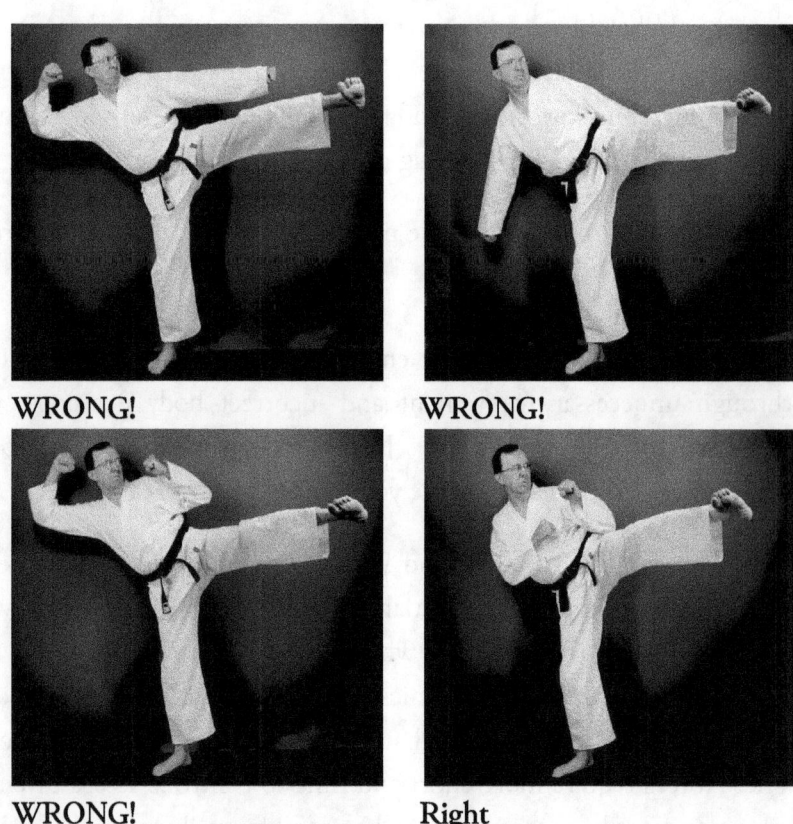

WRONG! WRONG!

WRONG! Right

Search For The Floor

When it comes to balance, the floor can be friend or foe. The floor is your friend any time that you know exactly where it is and your orientation to it. Many martial art styles incorporate foot movement that keeps the moving foot in light contact with the floor. This tactile feedback facilitates fluid control of balance as your body has two reference points with which to orient itself.

Making It Happen

This can be easily done without anyone noticing and without impairing your movement in the slightest. Simply extend your toes very slightly toward the floor and continuously touch lightly as you move. Your steps and foot movements should be smooth sliding motions rather than steps that take your foot well above the floor where you're in less control of your balance.

Strength And Stamina

Physical strength plays a large part in balance, especially static balance. That doesn't mean you must be overly muscular to effect exceptional balance. In lady's gymnastics, tiny and slightly built gymnasts exhibit seemingly superhuman feats of balance routinely. Persistently performing the training exercises listed below will adequately develop the muscles needed to greatly improve your balance.

Stamina is important to balance as well. Everything becomes difficult when you are exhausted. Ensure that you are working cardio appropriate for your martial art style to develop adequate stamina to maintain peak ability. Poor balance places additional demands on your stamina while superior balance reduces the demands on your stamina.

A Different Way To Kick

This kicking technique is for sparring and competition only. It facilitates speed and mobility but is not useful for delivering power. I use this style of kicking to enable myself to move in any direction at any time. Or, I can choose to not move at all. I can kick with full speed and extension, and then rechamber and place my foot back on the floor anywhere I want. That's because I don't move my center of gravity with the kick so that I maintain my balance. I can kick to the head and then move forward, sideward, angular, back, or just stay where I am. My decision to move, or not, is delayed as long as needed to take advantage of the situation as it unfolds. This gives me a tremendous tactical and speed advantage.

Kick without committing your center of gravity. Of course, there are thrusting and lunging kicks that require full commitment of your center of gravity in order to deliver full power with full body involvement. I'm referring here to kicks that don't have that requirement, such as snapping kicks, harassment kicks, kicks that set up another technique, kicks for reduced contact sparring, and any kick that derives its power from speed rather than commitment of body momentum. It is extremely common to see even black belts moving their center of gravity forward with every single kick. The kick is delivered, and rather than rechambering, the leg remains extended and the foot takes a nearly longitudinal path directly to the floor. This is an awkward and very slow process. It leaves you off balance and fully committed to forward movement. Throw a couple of these at a skilled opponent, and you will regret throwing a third one.

Spinning kicks suffer from a similar problem as they are typically executed. As the foot returns to its position behind you, your body and your center of gravity, shifts backward with it. Instead, maintain your center of gravity right where it is and extend your leg backward to place your foot into position. You will know that you are doing it right if you can stop with the kicking foot an inch off the floor and still maintain your balance without adjusting your torso. You should be able to stop fully at any point during the kick, or during the rechamber motion. See "Learn To Spin First, But Differently" (page 79).

You might be thinking you kick like this every time you kick in line drills. That is rarely the case. Although you are maintaining your position during your kicking practice, you are typically rechambering and returning to a predictable position and stance. Typically, your center of gravity will shift backward during the return to your starting position. This is very different than maintaining full control of your balance throughout the entire kick.

NOT Making It Happen

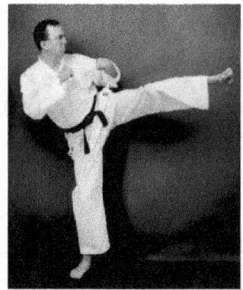

A typical kick has been executed. Everything looks fine at this point. The hands are well chambered and balance is good.

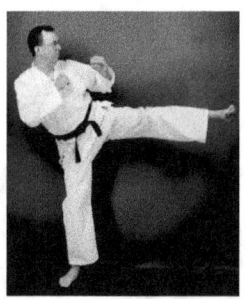

Something is going wrong. The foot is beginning to lower but the leg is still fully extended.

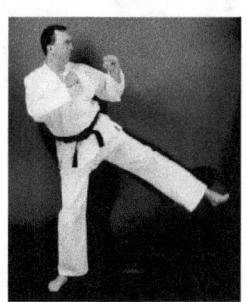

Now we're in disaster territory. The leg is still straight, the foot is dropping straight to the floor, and the body is committed to forward motion. There is no hint of a leg chamber.

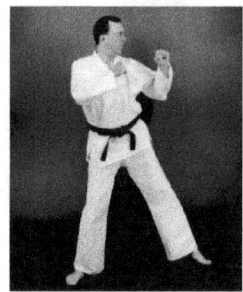 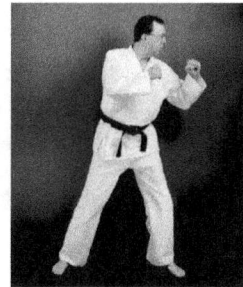

And, there it is. The foot clumps to the floor and the body moves forward at the mercy of uncontrolled momentum.

Making It Happen The Right Way

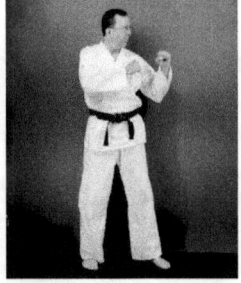
Ready to go.
Balance is perfect.

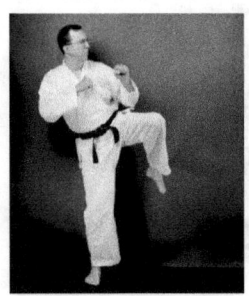
The kick starts.
Solid balance.

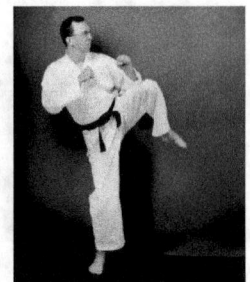
Deep chamber.
Solid balance.

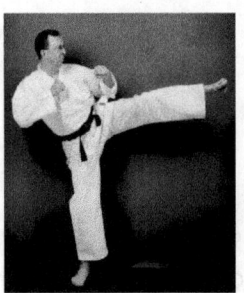
Typical kick.
Solid balance.

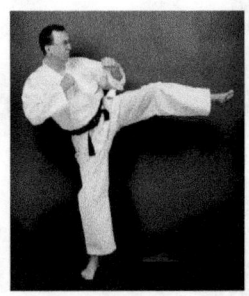
Rechambering.
Solid balance.

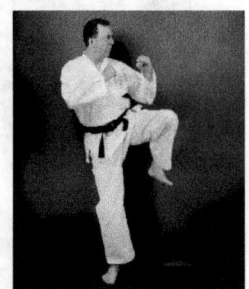
Back in chamber.
Solid balance.

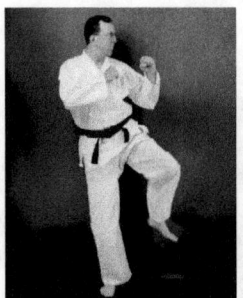
Returning to stance.
Solid balance.

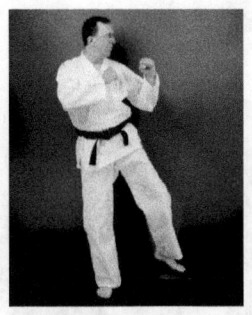
Almost back.
Solid balance.

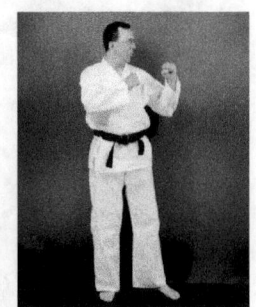
Back in stance.
Solid balance.

TRAIN IT

What is easy... do.
What is difficult... do more.

!!! WARNING !!!

To improve your balance, you need to push your limits. That can be dangerous as falls are not only possible, they're probable. Wear protective gear, especially headgear. Work on a padded surface. Have a capable partner ready to spot you. Work progressively and don't take chances.

Adapt These Training Exercises

These exercises are guides. You should adapt the concepts to your martial art style. Whenever possible, make the exercises mimic your martial art style. The most important thing is that you make them a deliberate part of your training and that you actively strive to improve.

Never Just Go Through The Motions

If you want to be exceptional, put in exceptional effort. During the entire process of every Train It, concentrate on what your body is doing to maintain your balance. Focus on your support foot and the parts of your foot that are in contact with the floor and where forces are being exerted by it and against it. Monitor the changes necessary in the position of your torso and every other part of your body. Learn what works and what does not. This focus is key to substantial improvement. Adjust, experiment, adapt, and learn what works and what doesn't. Never just practice. Make balance a deliberate pursuit.

How To NOT Train Balance

To improve our balance, we need to put ourselves in situations that place greater demands on our ability to balance. So, it seems logical that the greater the demand, the more benefit we will gain. If we train while standing on an unsteady or uneven surface, performing on stable and level ground will be a piece of cake. Right? Well, no.

This kind of training is very popular in many sports. The problem that coaches and trainers have discovered has to do with the motor engrams that you learned about in Chapter 4. You end up developing motor engrams for the uneven or unstable surface instead of ones that you will be using in performance. You will achieve better, and more applicable results, if you train in the conditions in which you plan to perform. You might look cool doing spinning kicks on a skateboard, but you aren't going to improve your fight speed as much as you would if you were kicking on a typical fight surface.

Train It #1
Do What You Do, But Do More

Just practicing martial arts develops balance. The problem is that development of balance is typically by default. I want you to make balance a focused, deliberate part of your training. Set aside time just for balance training. This doesn't mean just time for balance exercises. Training exercises are great, but more importantly, set aside time for your typical training with an emphasis and focus on balance during that training.

Train It #2
Broom Balancing

Broom balancing is something that I started doing just for fun in the mid-80s. At the time, I was doing a lot of kicking. One day I picked up a broom and balanced it on my foot. I kept doing it and quickly found that my kicks were improving substantially. I very rapidly developed much better balance, control, accuracy, power, and speed. I found it to be an excellent training exercise for developing foot-eye coordination as well. This is the exercise that I credit more than any other for the balance skills that have carried me for the past 37 years.

Balance

I once wrote an article for *Tae Kwon Do Times* magazine entitled, "Balance: The Foundation of Technique" that featured this exercise. It appeared in the May 1996 issue.

At first, this exercise may appear silly. Don't judge it by its appearance. This is a very powerful exercise with tremendous payoff for very little effort, no matter what martial art you practice. This exercise will greatly increase your static and dynamic balance. You will develop much greater fine control of your feet. You will develop much greater foot-eye coordination, which is something that we rarely train.

This exercise comes close to breaking my "no drills" rule. If done correctly though, it's still practical. Here is how to ensure that this exercise yields results that translate into real performance:

- *Use a very light-weight broom. This will limit the effects of added weight at the end of your leg. Added weight can enlist different muscle groups at different force levels than typical.*
- *Lift the broom into a position that is very similar to your kicking chamber.*
- *Use motions that are very similar to your normal kicking motion.*
- *Keep your body position as close as possible to your typical kicking position.*
- *Remember for balance, we are training the support leg more than the kicking leg.*

How it's done:

1. Obtain a lightweight broom.
2. Turn the broom upside down and place the end of the broomstick at the point where the base of your big toe and index toe meet (Fig. 10).
3. Turn the head of the broom perpendicular to your foot. This position makes balancing easier. You can alter this later as you gain proficiency.
4. Fix your eyes on the head of the broom.

5. Slowly raise your foot (the one that the broomstick is resting on) off the floor while still steadying the broom with your hands (Fig. 11). In the beginning, hold onto a chair or other stable object with one hand if necessary.
6. Adjust your support foot, leg, and center of gravity until you are stable. Your support leg's knee must be slightly bent.
7. Move the lifted foot in an effort to balance the broom while continuously loosening your grip on the broom head (Fig. 12).
8. Continue to keep your eyes fixed on the head of the broom. This is the easiest way to maintain control.
9. Practice until you no longer have need of holding to anything for assistance (Fig. 13).
10. Practice until you can balance the broom without the use of your arms for ballast and without need of support (Fig. 14, 15 and 16).
11. Work both legs.

When you become comfortable balancing the broom, increase the difficulty:
- Add vertical movement of your lifted foot by raising it up and down.
- Add side and circular movement of your lifted foot.
- Combine vertical, side, and circular movement of your lifted foot.
- Begin bouncing on your support foot.
- Add side, forward, backward, and circular movement of your support foot.
- Add difficulty by putting your hands behind your back.
- Add difficulty by substituting a bo staff in place of the broom. With less weight at the top, you will find the bo staff more difficult to balance.

Balance

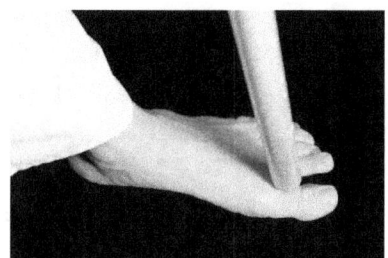

Fig. 10

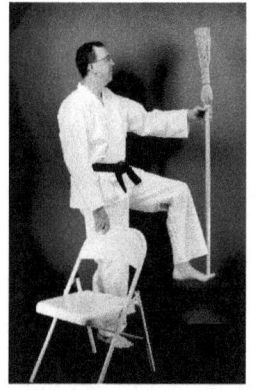

Fig. 11

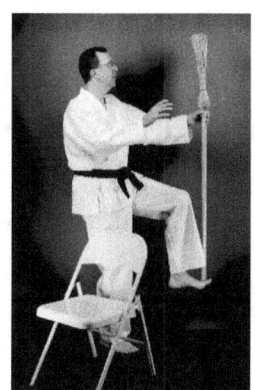

Fig. 12

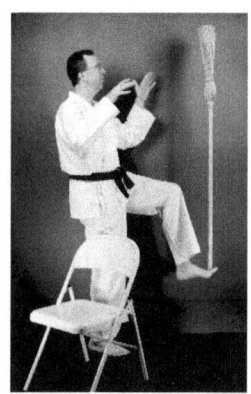

Fig. 13

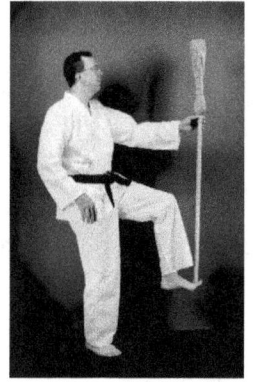

Fig. 14

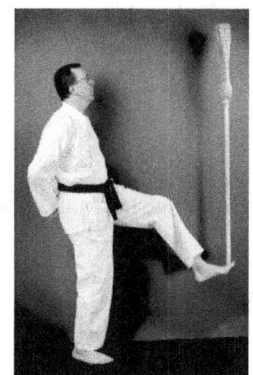

Fig. 15

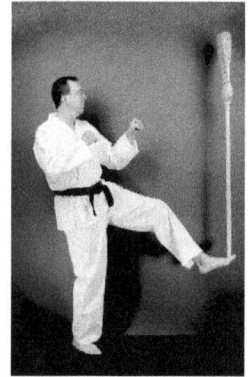

Fig. 16

Train It #3
Slow Kicking

This is a very effective exercise for anyone, not just styles that emphasize kicking. Even if you've never been trained in kicking, just extend your leg in place of the kicking motion.

1. Stand in a shallow fighting position (Fig. 17).
2. Keep your hands chambered. Extend your arms for a moment if you must, but as soon as you regain your balance, rechamber.
3. Chamber your selected kicking leg slowly. Ensure that it is a full, deep chamber (Fig. 18)
4. Hold the chamber for five to ten seconds.
5. Extend the kick slowly kicking at shin level (Fig. 19).
6. Hold the kick at full extension for five to ten seconds.
7. Rechamber slowly (Fig. 18).
8. Again, hold the chamber for five to ten seconds.
9. Extend the kick slowly kicking at knee level (Fig. 20).
10. Hold the kick at full extension for five to ten seconds.
11. Repeat the process by moving each kick up six inches higher than the previous kick. Stop when you reach the highest point at which you can kick comfortably and with proper form (Fig. 21 and 22).
12. Repeat the process in reverse.
13. Repeat for the opposite leg.
14. Repeat for different kicks or leg positions (if not trained in kicking).

When you become comfortable, increase the difficulty:
- Keeping your hands behind your back to reduce dependence on your arms for ballast when kicking.
- Close your eyes. *Ensure that you are in a safe area as you can easily fall. Having someone spot you is highly recommended.*
- Increase the speed of the movements.

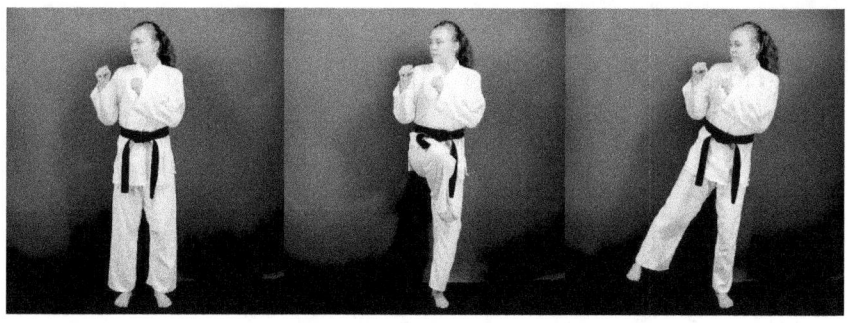

Fig. 17　　　　Fig. 18　　　　Fig. 19

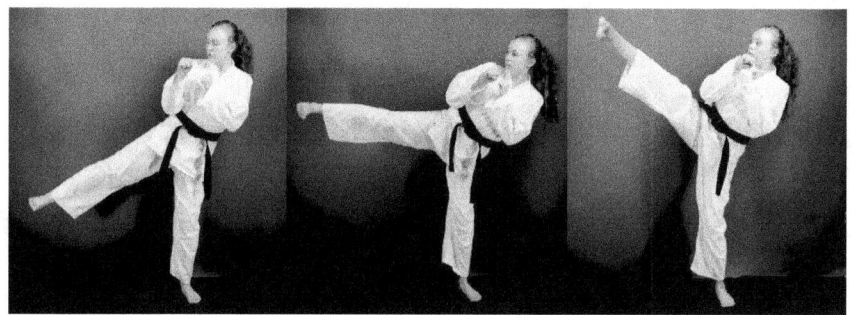

Fig. 20　　　　Fig. 21　　　　Fig. 22

Notice the absence of an exaggerated support foot pivot.

Train It #4
Hands Behind Your Back, For Everything

This is an easy exercise to adapt to your specific art. It is also extremely effective. Simply put your hands behind your back during your training. The goal is to become less dependent on the ballast provided by your arms and to improve the ability of your lower body to facilitate balance.

Here are a few examples:
- Forms practice – Forego hand techniques and complete all of the form possible with your hands behind your back.
- Sparring – With a firm agreement with your sparring partner, evade and advance without the use of your hands and arms. Keep them in chamber lest you develop some bad habits.
- Kicking practice – Stationary kicks, kicks on a heavy bag, kicks

with forward, lateral, and angular movement, and kicks on focus targets.
- Footwork training.
- Any training that you can safely execute without the use of your hands and arms.

Train It #5
Battle Balance

I like to keep training as relative as possible. The balance that is most important for a martial artist is the dynamic balance required to transition from one body position to another during an encounter with an opponent. Most of the forces working against your balance come in two varieties. First are forces are of your own creation that are at least somewhat predictable. The remainder of the forces are external and primarily caused by your opponent and the environment. Training to maintain balance in the face of unpredictable external forces requires creating unpredictable forces.

You need a very trusted and capable partner for this exercise. It is imperative that you and your partner understand the goals involved. The two of you must discuss, understand, and agree to reasonable limits. Failure to do so can result in serious injury.

How It Works

This exercise is fairly simple in design. Your training partner grips a large body shield with both hands. While you shadow spar, your partner hits and pushes you with the shield in an effort to force you off balance. The pushes and hits must be enough to interfere with your balance, but controlled enough to not cause you to fall or suffer injury.

Your partner is to use the shield to push you from multiple angles. The pushes must be unpredictable and timed to take advantage of moments that you are vulnerable to loss of balance such as during rechambering of kicks, stance changes, or during execution of power strikes and kicks.

Balance

Your partner's movements and timing should mimic that of an opponent minus the actual attacks. Keep it as realistic as possible.

The absence of the need to defend yourself affords you the freedom needed to work on your dynamic balance in real time. Pay close attention to your stances, stance transitions, upper body position and commitment, arm positions, and your balance recovery movements. Your job is the learn to adapt and correct in real time while not only maintaining your balance but also your composure and focus.

Pushes from behind can be very dangerous and are not recommended.

Train It #8
Slow Motion Everything

Simply slow down your regular training. This could be line drills, forms practice, kicking, hand strikes, blocks, take-downs, take-down defense, etc. It really doesn't matter. Just slow it down enough to force you to work at maintaining your balance.

This is not only a good workout and good balance practice; it is a great time to study and concentrate on each part of your body involved in maintaining your balance. But, don't just observe. Experiment and alter your positions and the routes that your limbs travel in order to become more efficient and to reduce the forces that work against your balance. Never just go through the motions. Constantly search for efficiency and better control.

Taking It To The Next Level

The Grappler's Advantage

Of the senses, touch is the fastest. Grappling arts train constantly for takedowns and takedown defense by being in constant contact with their opponent. Not to mention that they use full force. Because there is an actual opponent, the training is completely unpredictable (excluding what you may have learned about your opponent in the past). This is such an integral part of the grappler's training that it becomes completely instinctive. This is a daily ritual for grapplers. It is why most of them are so darned difficult to take down, and why they can typically take a non-grappler to the ground at will. Since it is very common for self-defense situations to go to the ground, stand-up fighters should add grappling to their training.

Making It Happen

If you are not interested in studying the grappling arts, at least add take-downs and take-down defense to your daily training. Find a competent instructor who will teach you and your training partner proper form. Then make this practice a part of your daily or weekly training routine. Train from the clinch and separated.

Don't Think About It

Developing skills to the point of subconscious proficiency is supremely important to martial artists. When one is subconsciously proficient, conscious thought is unnecessary. This is when speed is at its peak. Nowhere is this more important than it is with your balance. This is because all of your other skills reside on the foundation provided by your balance. If you are thinking about your balance, then you are not thinking about your opponent. This distraction can be devastating.

Always On

Balance should not be something that you turn on and off. You should train to make exceptional balance a part of you. This is much easier than you might think. Just make your balance practice a part of everything that you do. When walking along a curb, step up and walk it like a balance beam. When waiting in line, slightly lift one foot off the floor. At home, flip the light switch with your toes. Think about your balance all day so that you don't have to think about it during your martial arts training, or when a self-defense situation manifests. Yeah, this sounds dumb, but it works. Speed happens when you can do things without thought. Make balance the norm rather than the exception.

Analyze It

I know that I'm repeating myself here, but it's that important. When you are working on your balance, you should stay conscious of your efforts. Pay very close attention to what works and what doesn't. That doesn't mean casual observation. Deeply analyze the tension in your foot, how much your knee is bent, your torso position, the position of your head, how your weight is distributed across your foot, how you move your body, etc. Always note what works and what doesn't, and constantly improve. Most martial artists just practice. If you want to dominate, go deeper and improve every time you train.

Video

Video yourself and search for any area that can be improved. As explained in Chapter 7, runners often have their stride analyzed in tremendous detail to improve their efficiency. These are runners who have excelled, and they still have their stride analyzed in search of improvement. That's because there is tremendous value in the process. Use every tool possible to improve.

6

Distance
Be faster without being faster.

REDUCING THE DISTANCE TO YOUR TARGET WILL get you there faster. You're instantly faster without moving any faster. It doesn't get much more simple than that, right? It is a simple concept, but implementation can be a little complex. Complex, but not difficult. Taking advantage of distance control can be an easy, as well as effective, way to gain speed. A few simple changes in your weapon utilization, and you can increase your speed even more. Take control of distance, and you can take control of your opponent. Control your opponent, and the fight is yours.

The Definition Of Speed For Martial Artists
"The time that elapses from perception to effective completion."

When The Light Turned On For Me

It was about a year before I received my first black belt when I became interested in tournament competition. One evening, I happened across a Professional Karate Association (PKA) bout on TV. I watched closely hoping that I would learn something. The jabs and lead foot kicks immediately caught my attention. These were techniques that were not taught in the very traditional school that I attended. It was immediately clear that they would give me a distinct speed advantage. How much more easy could it be? Just strike with something closer to your target. The kicks were the most interesting to me. The PKA fighters were not only kicking with the lead leg, they would also close distance as the kick was executed by moving their entire body forward during the chamber motion of the kick. They would sometimes advance four feet or more. As I watched closer, I could see that distance control was as much a part of their strategy as their strikes and kicks. It was simple and very complex at the same time.

I started working on emulating those kicks and strikes that night in my living room. The next day I put them to work in my training. At first, I was soundly scolded by my master instructor. I still couldn't help but slip in a few lead techniques here and there. For some reason, he soon backed off, and just let me go. This was the beginning of my study of the relationship between distance and speed.

Distance Is Three Dimensional

In terms of speed, we are typically most concerned with distance as it relates to forward and rearward movement, as most attacks and defenses happen in those directions. Most beginners constantly retreat straight backward. This is extremely detrimental to your speed because it does nothing to improve your counterattack distance. And, it often forces you to stop your rearward momentum before effecting a counter. Straight rearward retreats allow your opponent to utilize their forward momentum to close distance easily, which gives away speed.

- **Lateral movement** for defense is much faster than straight-line movement. Avoiding an attack can be effected with much less movement by simply stepping slightly to the left or right. This leaves you within distance to quickly execute a counterattack.

- **Angular movement** is excellent for speed and distance control. Angular attacks can be some of the most effective and some of the most confounding for your opponent because few martial artists utilize angular movement. A confounded or confused opponent is always a slow opponent. Using an advancing angular movement to avoid an attack will simultaneously shorten your distance for executing a counterattack. You close distance to more easily execute a counterattack and avoid an attack in a single movement.

- **Vertical movement** is very important for speed as well, primarily for defense. Misusing vertical movement, like having your head in a lower position, can enable your opponent to execute a faster knee strike or uppercut.

When using lateral or advancing angular movement for defense, you MUST ensure that you are not moving into your opponent's attack which will give away both speed and power to your opponent.

Take Control Of Distance

Control of distance is control of the fight. Control of distance is also control of speed. This holds true in sparring and in self-defense. Every choice you make has advantages as well as disadvantages. How you control distance is primarily up to you and will be based on your experience, skillset, situation, and your martial art style. Below are some examples that will guide you to an understanding of distance control.

Reducing the distance that you must travel will effectively increase your speed by reducing the time needed to effectively complete an attack or counter. Conversely increasing the distance that your opponent must travel will reduce your opponent's speed, effectively increasing your

Distance

speed, by increasing the time required for your opponent to effectively complete an attack or counter.

Making It Happen

As you read the points below, constantly think in terms of your martial art style. Focus on how the concepts can be applied to your specific martial art style and your specific body to shorten distance wherever possible in order to effect greater speed.

Move Your Weapons Closer

The easiest way to increase speed by controlling distance is to move your weapons closer to your target or use a weapon that is already closer. A lead hand jab will reach its target faster than a reverse punch simply because it has less distance to travel. This will be at the cost of power (more on this below). Lead foot kicks reach their target faster than trailing foot kicks. Again, there can be a loss of power. However, many lead foot kicks can deliver devastating power.

Be aware that moving any part of your body closer to your opponent can make you more vulnerable to attack, especially by grapplers. A hand positioned closer to your opponent can be controlled by your opponent to effect a takedown and/or joint control. It can reduce your technique selection as well. Much of this is style and situation specific.

Making It Happen

If you don't have lead techniques in your arsenal, add them. If you have them but seldom use them, train to use them more effectively. If necessary, switch your stance from orthodox to southpaw or vice versa to put them to use. Switching stances often in a match is an effective strategy for several reasons. Like we're discussing here, it can move a weapon closer to your opponent. Switching stances can have the added advantage of frustrating your opponent, which is great for slowing your opponent. An ambidextrous fighter is a versatile fighter. A versatile fighter has more opportunity to be a fast fighter.

For sparring and competition, you have no better lead technique than the jab (or some would say the backfist), not so much for self-defense though. Boxers often win or lose by the jab. The jab is an excellent weapon of harassment, and there is no better setup hand technique for power punches.

Use A Longer Technique

If starting from the same position, a longer technique will reach your target faster. A hand strike with an extended hand or a kick with an extended foot will be slightly faster than techniques with a closed hand or a kick using heel contact. Those few inches can easily make all the difference. Of course, using a technique that is effective is of primary importance. Using a longer technique is more effective the greater the distance you are from your opponent. This is even more true if you have a reach advantage. When fighting very close to your opponent, these advantages diminish.

Making It Happen

Hands - Extended hand techniques are not useful for sparring and competition. Extended fingers are typically not legal because they pose a serious injury risk for both fighters. They can be useful for self-defense for eye and throat attacks. There are some downsides though. Extended fingers require extreme accuracy, which is nearly impossible in a self-defense encounter. Your fingers will probably be seriously injured as well, but if you're attacking the eyes or throat, your attacker will get the worst of it. Injured fingers are a small price to pay to quickly stop a violent attacker.

Feet – Extended feet are great for sparring and tournament fighting but not so effective for self-defense. For sparring and tournament fighting, nearly any kick can be executed with an extended foot to gain a few valuable inches. My spinning hook was my breadwinner for years. My fully extended foot often made all the difference and allowed me to throw with full speed without impacting with force that would get me disqualified. Extend your foot at the last moment. Contraction of the calf muscles creates tension that will slow your movement. Extended feet are not nearly as useful for self-defense because it's more difficult to transfer power into the target. A heel or knife edge impact is more effective. An extended foot can be useful for a thrusting kick to the lower abdomen with a ball of the foot impact or a groin strike with an instep impact.

Use Your Opponent's Forward Motion

Your opponent's forward motion shortens the distance for you by closing the gap. Because your converging speeds are cumulative, the distance closure is very fast as well, which adds even more speed.

Taking advantage of your opponent's forward motion is very dependent on accurate timing. Reading your opponent's habits can aid in timing forward movement especially if you pick up on a habit that is very predictable. Everyone is predictable if observed long enough. Using your opponent's forward motion can add to your power too. This is also due to the cumulative speeds of you and your opponent (if you're converging), which effectively increases the impact speed.

Attack A Closer Target

Viable targets include anything that is close and vulnerable. Shortening the distance shortens the time to effective completion. That makes you faster. Potential targets are the lead leg, the leading side of the ribcage, any portion of the body that comes closer to you during an attack, or loss of balance, etc.

The distance is shortened even more when you attack with a lead weapon. For harassment, during sparring and competition, I recommend striking the hands whether gloved or not. Slapping the hand works well if not gloved. If your opponent tends to take a step during attacks, ensure that you attack the advancing side to shorten the distance for the attack as well as to increase power by taking advantage of your opponent's forward motion.

Increase Distance For Your Opponent

There are countless ways to increase distance for your opponent. For self-defense, this can mean anything from running away to putting obstacles between you and your opponent. For sparring and competition, this means use of footwork, body position, and body movement. Being able to read your opponent is very valuable when choosing a method by which to increase distance for your opponent when sparring or competing. Knowing what your opponent is going to do, tells you where you need to go.

Making It Happen

Here are just a couple of examples. If you have a reach advantage, use it by staying in your range while staying just out of your opponent's range. As your opponent delivers a reverse punch, lean your torso away and deliver a side kick into the midsection. This extends the distance necessary for your opponent to reach your head and reduces the distance needed to deliver your kick because of your opponent's advance and lean toward you.

Distance, Power, And Accuracy

Often gaining speed, through distance control, is a tradeoff between speed and power. Reducing distance to gain speed reduces your ability to generate power as this leaves you with less distance to accelerate toward your target. Shortening the distance sometimes involves using lead techniques which are already positioned closer to your target. Lead techniques are typically less powerful as they tend to rely on the strength of the striking limb alone rather than using the power and mass of the entire body.

This loss of power makes target selection and technique selection very important. If your situation results in a loss of power, a softer, more vulnerable target should be selected. For example, in a self-defense situation, a lead hand strike may be less powerful but still devastating if it is targeting the throat or some other fragile part of the body. Power can be increased by using your opponent's advance to reduce distance. Your opponent's forward motion will add to your speed, as well as your power, as the two opposing forces and movements meet.

Timing becomes more critical than usual. You must expend power at the proper distance which requires accurate assessment of your opponent's movement. Expending power at the wrong distance renders your speed ineffective. This means that you must accurately compensate for your opponent's motion as it adds or subtracts from your motion. This kind of skill is acquired only by experience and lots of it.

Reading Your Opponent For Distance Control

For example, you begin to expect lead hand jabs from your opponent. Typically, a lead hand jab is accompanied by a small shift forward as well as a slight lean forward. Both of these factors reduce the distance to your opponent. At the instant, the lead hand begins to move you initiate a lead foot side kick with a slight lean of your torso backward. A small slide forward with the momentum of the kick will increase your effectiveness. Your kick should take the most direct route possible to your opponent's midsection. If your opponent has been telegraphing the jab, you should initiate the kick at the instant that you perceive the telegraph.

Move Your Faster Side To The Front

Most martial artists have a faster side and a more powerful side. This is where learning to fight ambidextrously can be a great advantage. When speed is needed more than power, like when wearing an opponent down with harassment type strikes, move your faster side to the front. When power is needed, switch stances if necessary. These types of choices are very personal and based on your skillset and body. Of course, you can add to your skillset through training. When using this approach, you must be very careful to not become predictable as this can negate any speed advantage you may otherwise have gained.

Striking Offense

For striking, hit the heavy bag, focus mitts, or whatever is appropriate to your desired fighting style. Have someone move your target so that the distance varies. Make it as unpredictable as possible. Be careful to protect your joints during misses. Do all of this with deliberate emphasis on controlling your distance and increasing your speed to your target. When you strike, pay very close attention to the distance at which your power is expended. You must deliberately work to expend your power into your target rather than short of it or beyond it. When your power is expended accurately, you are in control of your distance.

Striking Defense

Get hit. You and a training partner need to put on heavily padded gear so that you don't need to be concerned about injury. Have your partner attack you. You will be on defense only. Deliberately concentrate on control of your distance and your opponent's distance. This should be repeated with multiple training partners and with varying fighting styles. Make the attacks as varied and unpredictable as possible.

With concern for injury out of the way, you can concentrate on improving your control of distance and speed. No predictable line drill will ever train you as well as working with a training partner who is moving at realistic speed and intensity. The main factor here is to remove the concern for protecting yourself so you can experiment and concentrate on distance and speed in order to improve.

Chambering Too Close To Your Body

Holding your hands in chamber too close to your body has many distance and speed disadvantages. I see this more with beginners who do this due to being nervous and unsure of themselves. Unfortunately, I see many experienced martial artists doing this as well. Often the

Distance

hands are held tightly against the body. These are just a few of the disadvantages of chambering to close to your body:

1. **Offensive distance** – The distance to your target is increased, which robs you of speed.
2. **Defensive distance** – Allows attacks to get closer to you before you can intercept them which again, is a speed disadvantage.
3. **Slower** – Holding your arms close to your body causes excessive tension in the biceps which are the antagonists for extension. That tension is difficult to overcome and will slow the extension of that arm.
4. **Mechanical disadvantage** – Tightly flexing the arms elongates the triceps and places the upper and lower arm in a position that requires more effort to initiate an extension, as when striking. This relates to the difference of effort required to execute a bench press starting with the bar laying on your chest, as opposed to starting with your arms at a 90-degree extension. Initiating movement is much easier at the 90-degree position.
5. **Easier for you to be harassed** - If hands are held high, they will be very close to your face. This makes it easy for your opponent to drive them into your face. This gives your opponent a great distance advantage.

Making It NOT Happen

A proper chamber is going to vary by style as well as situation. There will be times that your chamber will be farther from your body, such as when effecting a takedown, or closer to your body, as when in a clinch. Conversely, there are no valid times to chamber with your hands against your body. While I can't give a proper chamber for every style, I can give you some basic rules:

- Keep the angle of your chamber (upper and lower arm) between 80 and 110 degrees.
- Keep your closest hand at least 6 inches forward of your chest.
- Use minimal bicep tension to maintain chamber position.
- During chamber, keep your hands below your chin.

- Don't clench your fists tightly. Tension reduces speed.
- Alter your chamber position to maintain situational advantage.

Footwork

Most stand-up martial artists severely neglect footwork. Lateral and angular movement is nearly nonexistent. Most move forward and backward as if on rails. To be very fast, you must be unpredictable and you must control distance from every direction. Too many styles and variables exist for me to be able to give a primer on footwork here.

I will tell you this much. Learn to move laterally and angularly with control of speed and distance. This alone will set you far apart from most martial artists and will facilitate a massive speed increase.

Stay light on your feet and on your toes, using constant movement. The idea is to be unpredictable, while always in an effective position. The more unpredictable you are the later your opponent knows what's coming. Being in position makes your attacks and defenses faster.

Using Distance To Counter Kicks

The most effective ways to negate a kick is to either move beyond the kick's reach or to advance well inside the kick's range. Moving beyond the kick's reach is effective but leaves you and your opponent in position to regroup and re-engage. You have avoided being kicked, but you've gained no tactical advantage. Timing your opponent's kick so that you end up inches away from your opponent while the kick is still extended can put you in position to land multiple hand strikes and can leave your opponent in poor position with only one foot on the floor. Keep in mind that advancing on a kick requires both timing and speed.

Making It Happen

- **Spinning kicks** - Advancing is extremely effective against spinning kicks. You must time your advance so that you move the instant that your opponent initiates the kick. Your goal is to be standing shoulder-to-shoulder with your opponent when the kick is extended. This is extremely frustrating for your opponent, and it puts you in a very dominant position.

- **Roundhouse kicks** – Advancing on a roundhouse kick can be a little tricky and risky. A lot depends on the type of roundhouse kick. Roundhouse type kicks can be delivered with a deep chamber and a straight-line approach or with a nearly straight leg in a long arc as in Muay Thai. The chamber can be with the lower leg parallel to the floor or perpendicular to the floor. In the case of the Muay Thai kick, advancing into the path of the kick can be very risky. If you choose to advance, you must advance fast enough to be inside of the knee to avoid the kick's power. You may choose to avoid the kick and then advance while it is continuing on its path past you. This is much slower but can still be a wise choice.

If your opponent utilizes a chamber with the lower leg perpendicular to the floor, a straight-line advance can be risky. This type of chamber is more vulnerable to an angular advance. Be careful because this type of chamber makes it easy for your opponent to stop or alter the kick at any point to change the attack. The chamber that is parallel to the floor is the easiest to advance on because it is slower, more telegraphic, offers little opportunity to change up, and takes a very predictable, easy to perceive path. On the other hand, it is very powerful so timing your advance correctly is critical.

- **Straight-line kicks** – An angular advance is the best approach for straight-line kicks. These kicks are very fast. They also make it easy for the kicker to change the kick's height and target even after the kick has been initiated. Straight-line kicks leave the kicker's center of gravity very stable and the hands free. All of that means that your best bet is to advance outside of the danger zone, which is anywhere directly in front of your opponent.
- **Typical kicks** - If your opponent is one of the crowd that kicks with extended and flailing arms, fails to rechamber, and has no

control of center of gravity, advancing becomes much easier. Just pick any moment that they are out of control and have your way with them.

High Kicks Cost Distance And Time

High kicks can be very effective for sparring and competition. In some styles, you receive two points for a head kick. Even so, there are serious distance and time considerations for high kicks.

- **High kicks lose distance** because of the angle at which they are delivered. When kicking to the abdomen (leg nearly parallel to the floor), you are afforded maximum reach. When you move your foot to head height, you cannot reach as far because of the steep angle of your leg. This means that you must be closer to your opponent to make contact. The result is that you have moved to where your opponent can get to you faster (with hands and abdomen kicks), but your technique (the high kick) arrives slower.
- **High kicks cost time** because it takes longer for your foot to travel from the floor to your opponent's head than it takes to get from the floor to your opponent's abdomen. It's simply a longer distance to travel. The extra travel requires more time. You must ensure that you have properly set up your opponent or properly read, and timed, your opponent to ensure that the opening will be there when your foot arrives.
- **Rechambering** requires more distance and time as well. For that reason, it is extremely important to keep your defenses up following execution of a high kick.

Get In Their Head And Shorten Distance In One Move

A lot of competitors carry their hands very high. This is because they don't like getting hit in the head. I dearly love sparring someone who does this. You can often easily hit their glove with a solid, straight punch and drive their own hand into their face. This is an extremely fast technique because the distance is greatly shortened by the thickness of your opponent's gloved hand. This technique has the added bonus of severely frustrating your opponent. This is not nearly as easy, or effective, against an opponent wearing MMA type gloves.

Stop Extending Your Arm To Measure Distance

Beginning martial artists are often instructed to extend their arm to measure distance. This is often done when lining up to practice self-defense. One hand is extended to set the distance to the opponent by touching their shoulder. Instructors have students do this for several reasons. The first is for safety as it reduces the possibility of inadvertent contact. It is also done to teach proper distance to maintain uniformity.

This practice is also common when striking a heavy bag or when breaking. No matter what the reason is, abandon this practice as quickly as possible. Do not let this become a habit. This is nothing but a crutch and an ineffective crutch at that. Do you extend an arm to measure when planning to use a doorknob to open a door? Do you extend an arm to measure the distance to the first step of a staircase before placing your foot on it? When you played kickball or soccer as a child did you extend an arm to measure the distance to the ball? No. All of that would be ridiculous, wouldn't it?

Your body is well equipped to measure distance intuitively. Conscious proprioception is your ability to be aware of your body position as well as the position of your body segments whether stationary or in motion. In other words, you know where your body is and where it's going. Proprioception is what enables you to touch your nose with your eyes closed. Use this system's ability and forego the measuring. You don't have time for it, you don't need it, and it has no practical relationship to fighting. Because some of the movements in martial arts are foreign and awkward for beginners, distance measurement may require a little practice, but you don't need to reach out and touch anything.

If your instructor tells you to do something for safety, then do it. Ask questions, but never do anything that reduces safety.

7

Efficiency

Master this and everything happens faster.

I DON'T CARE HOW FAST YOU MOVE YOUR HANDS OR feet if your movement is inefficient you are slow. This is another subject that is about as exciting as plain oatmeal. You need to decide if you want sugared-up garbage cereal or if you want what's good for you. Efficiency is imperative for speed. Your every movement must be purposely made to accomplish your goal in the shortest time possible. Sugared-up flashy techniques and useless wasted movement will destroy your speed. Even minor changes in your movement can yield significant increases in speed. Eliminating the big inefficient habits, that most of us have, can massively increase your speed.

Traditional Martial Arts

I respect, practice, and enjoy traditional martial arts for many reasons, but efficiency is not one of them. Traditional martial arts, as taught in most schools (not all) are massively inefficient, especially at the lower ranks. It's common for many, if not all, techniques to be taught to beginners and lower ranks as very mechanical, exaggerated movements delivered from exaggerated impractical stances.

There are many reasons for this approach that include conditioning and coordination development. Often, it is for illustrative purposes. The thinking is that it makes the technique easier for a beginner to understand and see the body mechanics involved in the technique. In some styles, it is simply the way things are done.

I strongly disagree though. I prefer to teach as close to correct form as possible from the beginning rather than spend time un-teaching and re-teaching later. For scientific proof of why this approach is seriously flawed, read the "Motor Engrams Master Class" starting on page 50.

Where Tradition Goes Seriously Wrong

As students move into the upper ranks, most instructors and styles will refine those inefficient, exaggerated techniques taught early on making them more practical, faster, powerful, and more efficient. Unfortunately, this is not always the case. I've seen many students cling to those exaggerated movements and even put them into use in sparring. It's scary to think that they may even try them for self-defense.

I'm not going to ask you to abandon your martial art style. I will ask you to objectively evaluate what you are doing to find ways to execute your techniques more efficiently, and therefore, faster. Use runners as an example. It is safe to say that anyone who competes in running probably knows well how to run. Heck, anybody can run. Right? Why then do Olympic and other elite runners use technology to evaluate, in agonizing detail, every component of their stride from the ground up? They use high-speed video, a myriad of measuring devices, and sophisticated computer analyzation to find every possible imperfection and inefficiency in their stride. Then, they work to eliminate those imperfections and inefficiencies through purposeful training. That is because even tiny improvements in efficiency can lead to more speed and effectiveness. If a runner is willing to objectively critique something as simple as the way that they run (it's actually not all that simple) then, a martial artist should be willing to examine their technique, regardless of how revered their style is.

No Need For Conflict

Most instructors will not permit you to make changes to traditional techniques, but that is of little concern. The need for efficiency is in sparring and self-defense. The traditional techniques found in forms, katas, and line drills are rarely executed in sparring or self-defense, so there is little chance for conflict. If you have a particularly strict instructor, you may need to do your training out of sight or even outside of your school. The speed gain will be well worth the trouble.

Your Job

It's going to be up to you to find your inefficiencies. There are so many highly varied styles that it is not possible to evaluate them all here. We are going to review a few very common inefficiencies here as examples to build your awareness of what to look for. Apply that knowledge very deliberately to all of your skillset.

You Need Help

Often, it is difficult to detect your own inefficiencies. It's safe to say that the Olympic runners in the example above all thought that they were running as efficiently as possible before they were evaluated because only accomplished, elite runners are selected for that kind of scrutiny. Those runners were already champions, so you can bet their coaches had already corrected everything they could in search of more efficiency. The runners themselves had done everything they could to become as efficient and fast as possible. And still, inefficiencies remained. You're going to need help too.

Making It Happen
- **Your Instructor** - Unfortunately, this is rarely the person to go to for help. Traditional martial art instructors are notorious for strictly conforming to what they've been taught. Then, there are

the so-called traditional schools, of the McDojo variety, where minute inefficiencies are of no concern and wouldn't be recognized if you were to hang a neon sign on them. Then, there are the instructors that can't see the forest for the trees just due to the massive time that they've spent doing things the way they do them. Some instructors will even be offended by the suggestion that there are inefficiencies in what they teach.

- **Video** - Video is a great way to evaluate any aspect of your performance. Video can be slowed for frame by frame inspection of body position, striking path, rechambering path, etc. Ensure that your video is shot in sufficient light and that the camera is held very steady. You should video situations that are as spontaneous as possible, preferably when you are under enough pressure to ensure that you are performing based on your training. Otherwise, you may consciously, or subconsciously correct your technique which may camouflage otherwise evident inefficiencies.
- **A Skilled Observer** - If you have the good fortune of having a training partner who understands your goals, have them observe your performance. Your observer must be completely objective with regard to style and your improvement. An observer who is more interested in preserving traditional style over efficiency is going to be of little help. A fellow competitor may or may not be your best ally either. After all, would you want to give your competition an advantage?

Most importantly, if you choose to use an observer, leave your ego in the locker room. Ego may prevent you from letting go of a cherished but inefficient, habit. Being corrected is never any fun, no matter how helpful it is. And, don't take their word for anything. Question everything because you may move the way you do because your body moves better that way. Everyone is different, and martial art techniques can be very personal. I don't pivot my support foot fully for side or roundhouse kicks. The range of motion in my hips is greater than for most people.

Correct me all you want, but I'm more efficient, in this case, my way. Base all of your changes on what works for you.

It's Not Complicated

Becoming efficient is not complicated at all. In fact, it's a little anticlimactic. All you need to do is execute your technique directly and then put whatever you used back where it can be used again in the most direct path possible. Notice that I did not say to put it back where it was because that may not be the most efficient place for it. Most of the time it is, but we need to always be ready for exceptions.

Take The Direct Route

When striking, take the most direct, and shortest, route to your target. When delivering a hand strike, your hand should travel the shortest distance possible with no straying off course. Most often that is a straight line to its intended target. That is always the fastest route.

There is an added bonus when using straight-line techniques. They are more difficult to perceive. To perceive, the approach of a fist traveling a straight line your opponent must detect the change in apparent size of the fist as it approaches. This is more difficult than detecting a fist that is traveling a path that has a component of lateral travel.

To add to the difficulty of perception, wear black gear. I believe that black gear is slightly more difficult to perceive than brighter colors. This works even better if you wear a black uniform so that your black gloves are cast against a black background.

It Doesn't Have To Be Straight To Be Direct

Of course, there are times that a looping or indirect technique is called for to overcome your opponent's defenses or to surprise your opponent. In those cases, you still should not deviate from the most direct, and therefore, most efficient path to your target for that technique. The straight-line route is always the fastest, but it is a poor choice if it reduces the effectiveness of the technique. If a looping approach is called for, make it an efficient loop.

Take A Direct Path Back To Chamber

This is where things most often go wrong and where the majority of bad habits will be found. Once a strike is completed, the striking extremity should be rechambered immediately. It is staggering to see how many martial artists, both amateur and professional, drop their hands after a strike. It's like firing a gun without chambering another round. As long as there is no ammunition in the chamber, you are effectively unarmed. Not to mention that a dropped hand typically leaves an opening that may as well have a welcome mat in front of it.

Rechamber Fast

Well, this is boring. Martial artists train to hit and kick things. We don't train for hours a day to learn how to put our hands in front of us. That's right. Most martial artists don't, but the fast ones do.

This is one of the most neglected areas of typical martial art training. There typically is little or even no mention of rechambering. This is like a basketball coach teaching shooting with no mention of rebounding. That's a great way to lose basketball games. Not rechambering fast is a great way to lose fights.

Not only must you rechamber immediately after a strike, the rechamber motion should be at least as fast as the strike. Striking fast and rechambering slowly is very inefficient and does nothing good for your speed. Practice rechambering with the same speed and intensity as you strike. Make rechambering fast a habit. Train rechambering as hard as you train your strikes. This one skill can increase your speed and effectiveness enough to take your speed to a whole new level.

Don't forget your kicks. Rechambering kicks fast is just as important, maybe even more important, because you need that leg to stand on for both kicks and strikes.

!!! Dang It! Get This Into Your Head !!!

Read the following paragraph as if I'm in your face screaming so loud that there's spit flying out of my mouth and my voice is cracking so bad that you think that I'm going to snap a vocal cord. Then, read it again.

RECHAMBER AS FAST AS YOU STRIKE! YOUR WEAPONS ARE USELESS IF YOU DON'T PUT THEM BACK WHERE THEY CAN BE USED. UNLESS YOU FINISH THE JOB WITH THE FIRST STRIKE 100 PERCENT OF THE TIME, RECHAMBERING IS JUST AS IMPORTANT AS STRIKING. TRAIN RECHAMBERING AS HARD AS YOU TRAIN STRIKING. TRAIN TO RECHAMBER WITH SPEED, AUTHORITY, AND EFFICIENCY. YOUR GOAL IS ALWAYS TO PUT THE STRIKING EXTREMITY BACK WHERE IT CAN BE USED AGAIN AS QUICKLY AS POSSIBLE. NEVER BE LAZY OR INEFFICIENT WHEN RECHAMBERING. RECHAMBER FAST DANG IT!

If You Still Don't Buy This Rechamber Fast Stuff

Just watch a couple of hours of professional fighting. Take your pick. MMA, Boxing, PKA, it doesn't matter. Just watch long enough to see a few knockouts. Start counting how many of them happen because of the losing fighter holding a hand low or dropping a hand after a strike. We're talking about professional fighters. Constantly, you see them drop a hand after a strike or just hang a hand in front of them. You know that it's just a matter of time, and then, they're on the canvas. If a professional fighter can't get away with it, you can't. If it gets them knocked out, it will get you knocked out. Rechamber effectively and do it fast.

Start 'Em Young

I tell kids to put their toys away. In this case, the toys are their hands, and the toy box is their chamber. Just like you put your toys away at home, put your toys away during your martial art training. And, just like at home, when you don't put your toys away, you get in trouble. At home, it's time out. Here, it's a glove to your head.

There Are Exceptions

There are always exceptions. For example, there are situations where the striking hand can be used for other purposes, such as grabbing before it is rechambered, so it makes sense to leave it extended. You may drop your hands in an effort to draw an opening or to set up a strike from your other hand. You may leave a hand extended to draw an opponent in for a takedown. These are not inefficient moves because they have a purpose.

The Chamber

All of this talk of rechambering fast is useless if you don't have an efficient and effective chamber position. Your chamber position will be heavily dependent on your martial art style and your personal style. Seek instruction from an accomplished instructor. Notice that I didn't say an experienced instructor, I said an *accomplished* instructor. Then, objectively and proactively evaluate your chamber to your own satisfaction. Your goal is to chamber where your assets are the most readily useful for both offense and defense.

Kicks

Kicks are one of the greatest sources of inefficiency in martial arts. This is seen much more often with amateurs. Most martial artists focus their kicking training on developing power. They kick the heavy bag over and over attempting to develop rib-cracking power. When they impact the bag, the striking foot will linger at its impact point and then drop directly to the floor. It will then be retracted back into place for another kick. In sparring, this translates to kicking and then dropping the foot to the floor with the leg extended like the kicking leg has a splint on its knee. Along with it comes the fighter's center of gravity in what equates to a lumbering step forward. Throw a couple of these against a skilled fighter, who is adept a reading and timing an opponent, and you will find yourself being counterattacked profusely.

Just as with hand strikes, rechambering is of utmost importance. The kicking leg must be retracted immediately to a place where it is useful for either another kick or for body support. During the kick and the rechamber, your center of gravity must be under your control, so that you move in the direction that is most efficient, rather than being forced to follow your kicking leg as it flops your foot to the floor.

For kicks to be efficient, you must control your body movement, center of gravity, and foot placement. Overcommitment of any kind requires time to correct. It requires motion and thought which are time intensive. Overcommitment is inefficient and slow.

Rechambering Kicks

Kicking line drills typically require kicks to be rechambered along the same path that they are executed on. You pick up the rear foot, chamber, kick, rechamber, and put the foot down again. You'd think that I would recommend this approach since I've spent so much of this chapter talking about rechambering on the shortest most direct path possible, but kicks are different.

So now, I've contradicted myself. I've spent most of this chapter telling you that the most efficient way to rechamber is to travel the same path that the technique took to get to its target, and now, I'm telling you that's not true for kicks. That's because your feet and legs are involved in much more than just kicking. They're also involved in your support

Efficiency

and footwork. Unlike a hand that can be extended and then rechambered to its original position, a foot may be involved in advancing, retreating, or firing off a second kick.

The rule for kicks is regardless of where your kicking foot needs to go when it has completed the kick, get it to that position as directly and quickly as possible. That may or may not be along the path the kick followed, but get it back into useful position as quickly as possible.

That means once your foot has contacted sufficiently with its target it gets withdrawn instantly. It doesn't linger at all. Get it to where you can use it immediately.

The Uncool Kick That Should Be Your Go-To

The front kick is a speed powerhouse that is extremely underutilized. It is arguably the fastest kick in your arsenal. Its only problem is that it's never on the cool kick list. The front kick has some very serious advantages over other kicks.

- **Extremely fast** - It travels the straightest, shortest, and most efficient path to its target of all kicks.
- **Dangerous** - It can deliver devastating power to very vulnerable targets.
- **Difficult to block** - Because of its straight-line approach to its target.
- **Difficult to perceive** – Its straight-line approach makes it more difficult to perceive than tangential kicks.
- **Less telegraphic** – The front kick can be delivered from nearly any body position with zero windup.
- **Close distance** – You can close distance with a lead or trailing foot front kick by either carrying your body forward with the momentum of the kick or simply taking a step forward.
- **Retreating** - It's easy to retreat while executing a front kick.
- **Superb counter kick** – A slight lean back during a front kick leaves your opponent's punch short of your head and your foot in

your opponent's belly.

- **Minimal hip rotation** - The front kick requires very little hip rotation, even for a thrusting kick, which means that you remain mobile in multiple directions.
- **Power settings** - The front kick can be delivered as a snapping kick, thrusting kick, or as a setup technique.
- **Harassment** – It is so quick and requires so little commitment that it makes a great harassment technique.
- **Simple** – Almost anyone can execute an effective front kick.
- **Setup** – The front kick is a great setup kick for other techniques because it is so easy to transition from a front kick to nearly any other technique.
- **Versatile targeting** – Effective from shin to chin.
- **Multiple striking surfaces** – Ball-of-the-foot, heel, or instep.
- **Very stable** – Because of its slight deviation from a stepping motion, it is very easy to maintain balance during a front kick.
- **Long reach** – The front kick is very long especially with ball-of-the-foot contact when the foot is fully extended forward.
- **Downside** – When using ball-of-the-foot or heel contact, the small striking surface of the front kick requires more accuracy than other kicks when kicking to the head or legs.

To be fast, a front kick must be executed properly. The front kick is sometimes taught with a very high chamber that nearly pauses before the kick is completed. To be fast, the chamber must be part of the kicking motion. Only chamber as much as is required to be effective. Snapping kicks require less chamber than thrusting kicks. Even thrusting kicks have minimal chamber depth required if your intent is to push more than impact. Chambering no more than necessary to be effective reduces the kick's travel time and therefore increases its speed.

Drop The Macho Junk

There seems to be some sort of machismo attached to poor fighting positions. Guys, in particular, like to drop their lead hand after a strike.

Some hold their lead hand low constantly. It's kind of like the street-tough bad guys in cop shows who hold their handgun turned on its side. They think it looks tough, but it's anything but effective. Let your opponent look cool. You opt for effective.

Hanging And Flailing Arms

Few things in martial arts look more pathetic than a fighter with arms hanging and flailing by their sides. Sure, Olympic Tae Kwon Do competitors get away with it. They typically keep their arms hanging by their sides using no chamber at all. This works well within the confines of their type of competition where kicks are emphasized. They still take some shots that they could have blocked. Some sport karate styles also keep their hands very low; even though, they tend to utilize more hand techniques. This is in part because often the action stops on each point, so counterstrikes are less important. I still disagree with it because it increases distance for strikes and blocks. Conversely in MMA and other full contact competitions, hanging and flailing arms can be suicidal. Even while sparring in most traditional schools, an effective boxer-like chamber or other effective chamber is necessary to be effective for offense and defense.

Bill "Superfoot" Wallace was famous during his Professional Karate Association (PKA) career for keeping his lead arm straight down over his lead leg. In his case, it was entirely on purpose. He had developed defenses using that position that were very effective for him. He utilized his shoulder and upper body movement to effect his defense. Given his 23-0 professional record at retirement, I think it worked for him. It helped that if you attacked that side you had to get past his famous lead foot, which was devastatingly fast and accurate.

For the rest of us, those hanging arms are an inefficient speed-killing disaster. Get your hands up and keep them there unless they're doing something effective (which can include dropping them to draw an opening). Learn a proper defensive position for your style and use it.

Stance

Every single thing that you are trying to do is dependent on your stance and your ability to transition from and to it. Your stance is very heavily dependent on your martial art style. If you are not in position to quickly and effectively execute your intended technique, you're inefficient and slow. The boxer-like fighting stance is typically the most efficient stance with some point competition styles (where a deep horse-riding type stance is effective) being exceptions. Cat stance, back stance, forward stance, horse-riding stance, and any stance with locked knees are never efficient stances for fighting and self-defense situations.

Leaving A Striking Limb Extended After A Strike

This is a very common habit and one that your opponent considers to be a gift. The strike is thrown, and the striking limb is left extended dangling in the air as if you've forgotten what you're doing. It's like a batter in baseball who stares at the ball after hitting it. Drop the bat and run, dummy. If it's a home run, great. If it's not, you may make it to first base. There are two primary problems caused by this:

- An extended limb is useless. You can only deliver another strike or execute a block if you rechamber. Rechambering means that you put it back where it can be used again.
- An extended limb is very useful to your opponent who will want to use it to control you, including taking advantage of the opening that it is creating.

Conditioning

Conditioning can win or lose a fight. No-one can be fast when they are fatigued. Efficient movement economizes your energy reserves simply by reducing the amount that you move. This pays off later in life. As I write this, I am 57 years old, and I'm in a period where time commitments do not permit me to dedicate myself to conditioning. My stamina has suffered as a result. When I move efficiently, I can perform well. When I don't move efficiently, I pay for it.

Touching Isn't Blocking

This is one of the most inefficient habits in martial arts. Beginners and black belts alike tend to reach out and touch incoming kicks that are going to fall short of connecting anyway. If there is not a good reason for your hands to move, they should remain right where they are most useful. Break this habit and break it now. Lowering your hand sufficiently to touch an incoming kick to the midsection leaves your head wide open.

You shouldn't be lowering your hands to block anyway. Attacks to your midsection should be blocked with your forearms leaving your hands in place to protect your head. This is efficient and fast.

Did You Really Need To Throw That?

Never throw anything without a reason. I've watched lower belts as well as seasoned black belts spar by throwing a constant barrage of kicks and punches. They look like windup toys that mindlessly flail about until they wind down. This is extremely inefficient; it wastes energy, and it lacks precision. Not to mention that it just looks ridiculous. That energy is needed for your speed. The precision is needed to effect speed and accuracy. Do everything you do with purpose.

Self-defense

Self-defense is a different world. Chambering immediately can provoke a fight when there might otherwise have not been one. In self-defense, we should focus on being ready more than chambering. The more deceptive the better. Being deceptive by not appearing to ready yourself for a fight, reduces provocation and preserves the element of surprise if you do choose to fight. If you do choose to fight, rechambering fast and efficiently becomes more important than ever.

Slipping And Evading

Slipping and evading are very efficient for defense. They require minimal movement and energy. If executed properly, you will simultaneously avoid attack and place yourself in position to counter-attack. Slipping and evading don't require the use of your hands, which leaves them instantly available for offense or defense.

Be careful when evading an attack. Moving too far or incorrectly will increase the distance required to execute a counter attack. Moving too far away can also make it easier for your opponent to reset or deliver a follow-up attack.

Slipping is the ultimate in efficient defense. Moving very slightly to allow your opponent's attack to just barely miss you requires very little effort or commitment of motion. Executing your counterattack while your opponent's attack is still extended leaves your opponent open and you in a very advantageous position. If your opponent's striking weapon is extended past you, that means that you are close enough to strike very quickly.

!!! WARNING !!!
Slipping strikes and blocking with abbreviated movements is very efficient, but also very difficult for others to see that you haven't actually been hit. This can sacrifice points in competition.

It Never Ends

This purpose of this book is not to evaluate your every technique. That is your job. A martial artist should be in a constant search for efficiency. Some call it a search for perfection. With the countless styles in existence, and the massive volume of techniques within those styles, this chapter could literally go on forever. For you, hopefully, it will.

8

Strength and Conditioning

You can't be fast when you're gassed.

FATIGUE IS AN EXTREME ENEMY OF SPEED. POOR conditioning will undo everything else in this book. If your body is poorly conditioned, you may still be able to move fast, but you won't be able to do so for very long. It's just not possible to be fast and exhausted at the same time. Moving fast is very taxing on your muscles and stamina. Ballistic movements can easily injure a poorly conditioned body. Balance, accuracy, timing, power, your mental game, and everything else suffers when you are tired. It is imperative that you maintain a well-conditioned body for maximum speed and effectiveness as well as for your safety.

Most Martial Art Schools Neglect Conditioning Good For Them

Get in shape on your own time. I'm a firm believer that your time in a martial art school should be used to learn martial arts, and how to effectively use what you've learned. Conditioning should be limited to a solid warm-up utilizing basic skills at the beginning of class and intense practice including sparring. An even better approach would be to require students to arrive early and warm-up on their own. This isn't because conditioning isn't important. It's because martial art training is serious business and should be treated as such. Burpees and aerobics have no place in martial art training. And, don't even get me started on stinking relay races. It's also because of how important conditioning is. There are far too many breaks in a typical martial art class to make it an effective conditioning workout. Conditioning should be a training session of its own.

Muscles And Speed

It is not necessary to be particularly muscular to be fast. In fact, as you've no doubt witnessed, fighters of smaller stature are typically faster than heavily muscular fighters. More important than quantity of muscle is having well-conditioned muscles. For speed, muscle conditioning is possibly even more important for heavily muscular fighters due to the extra mass that they must move.

There is a minimum requirement though. I was very skinny and sickly when I walked into my first martial art class. I was small, weak, and slow. A couple of years later I was still very small, but I was much better conditioned. My speed had improved substantially due only to my improved conditioning. At that point, I had added no more than five pounds to my frame. I would often poke fun at myself for being so skinny. My friends would tell me that I didn't need a lot of muscle to be fast. I would reply, "Yeah, but I at least need enough muscle to move my bones." That's all in fun, but there's a point here. Just being small isn't enough for speed. You must be well conditioned too.

Strength Training And Weight Training

Now I'm diving into major debate territory. There's very little consensus on either of these subjects. Is strength training necessary for speed? Will weight training help or hurt your speed? Do a little research, and you will find so many different opinions that you'll give up martial arts and take up knitting.

Strength and Conditioning

Let's look at it logically. If you pick up a paper cup, you can move it very fast. If you pick up a gallon jug of milk, you can't move nearly as fast. If you were strong enough to make that jug of milk feel as light as the paper cup, you could move it just as fast as the cup. The logical conclusion is that strength helps with speed.

For striking, the only thing that you need to pick up is the limb that you're moving and maybe some protective gear. Once you have developed the strength to move all of that as fast as you desire, anything else is gravy.

Grapplers, arguably, are more dependent on strength than strikers. Technique is paramount for being effective, but strength can still provide tremendous advantages. Full body strength training in their training regimen is a must. For speed, they must be mindful of the same potential for problems as strikers.

Problems You May Encounter
- If you add mass without adding proportional strength, you will reduce your strength to weight ratio, which will essentially add milk to the jug you're moving. Lifting your own body becomes the effort that slows your movement.
- If you weight train improperly (using very abbreviated movements), you can reduce your range of motion, which will inhibit your speed.
- Weight training involves tremendous muscle tension. I've seen some martial artists become so focused on strength and weight training that the tension used in their lifting became habit. That tension greatly reduced their ability to relax their muscles, which is imperative for moving fast.

Making It Happen
- Gain enough strength to easily move your limbs at full speed.
- When strength training, use full range movements that do not condition you to a reduced range of motion. Be careful to not

lock your joints as this may cause injury.
- If you add mass, add and maintain proportional strength.
- When strength training, be vigilant about maintaining your ability to relax your muscles.
- Ensure that you maintain your flexibility in the areas that you are strength training.
- Include your core, shoulders, and lower body in your strength training. Your strength must remain proportional throughout your body. This goes for strikers as well as grapplers.
- ALWAYS use proper form when strength training.
- Avoid isolating muscles. Always train for synergetic strength improvement that translates to your speed goals.

Training Before Competition

It amazes me how many coaches, instructors, and competitors will continue a full training regimen right up to competition time. There's nothing like keeping yourself fatigued right up until show time. You can't possibly be fast when you are still recovering from training.

Drop to maintenance level before a competition. When to drop your training level, depends on your current condition, your particular training regimen, and your typical time needed for recovery. The point is to show up at the competition in peak condition and at peak recovery. This might require some test runs to get it just right, so get started now. Keep a journal of your condition in the days after dropping your training to maintenance level.

Even if you're feeling good, I still advise one to two days of no training right before a competition. You can't be fast with a fatigued body.

Warm Up

NEVER workout or train without warming up first. That warmup is an absolute must for speed training. Speed training is very strenuous and offers plenty of opportunity for injury, especially if your body is not prepared for the activity. Before training, always warm up with light cardio appropriate for your style and targeted at the muscles that you intend to train. Do not warm up with strenuous exercises that will fatigue your muscles. Speed training will push your limits. Do not fatigue your muscles right before training them for increased speed performance.

Don't Spar For Stamina

I bet that line got your attention. There is no doubt that sparring is a great workout. No exercise routine is going to provide the fight specific workout that sparring does. That's because the physical demands on your stamina and general conditioning are much greater when someone is hitting back. Even more important is the fact that no exercise routine can simulate the effects of the adrenalin and mental stress that you face when actually sparring. So, it is essential that you spar hard enough and long enough to gain the conditioning and mental preparedness that only sparring provides. Your speed depends on it.

The problem is that there are too many breaks in typical sparring. If you are a skilled and experienced martial artist, you have found many ways to recover and rest during lulls in the action. You've no doubt learned to create those lulls when needed. These skills are essential, but they don't translate into an effective stamina workout. Your stamina workout should be structured so you can ensure that you are progressing. You can log the minutes that you're in the ring, but you can't gauge how much effort you expended. Then, there is the matter of each opponent placing different demands on your sparring time. That's why I prefer something like the routine described below.

HIIT The Gym For More Speed And Stamina

This is a good time to re-read the disclaimer at the beginning of this book. HIIT is extremely physically demanding. Get your doctor's approval before attempting a HIIT session.

High-intensity interval training (HIIT) has been the subject of several studies that have made news headlines over the past few years. The attention-getting fact is that, according to the studies, a very short HIIT regimen can deliver the same health benefits, including cardiorespiratory improvement, as much longer traditional workouts. So, HIIT appears to be very efficient and effective.

HIIT does have a dark side though. HIIT, if done right, is brutal and, in my opinion, a little dangerous. Especially so, for those who are not already in good physical condition. That is because the high-intensity portion of the workout is typically done at maximum effort.

The next problem is that the jury is still out. While there are many studies that support HIIT and sprint-interval training (SIT), which is very similar, there are some critics as well. The debate is so intense at the time of this writing that it is difficult to draw an acceptable conclusion. Still, I believe that HIIT holds promise for speed training.

- The workouts are formatted in short intervals of extremely high-intensity activity followed by longer intervals of moderate activity. This relates well to fighting whether for competition or self-defense where brief flurries are followed by less intense periods.
- The high-intensity segments of a HIIT workout are perfect for very fast movement because they are all-out sprints using everything that you've got. Again, that plays perfectly into speed training as well as fighting.
- HIIT also gets it over with quick. If you have a demanding schedule, HIIT is a workout that is easy to fit in. HIIT also does double duty by working speed and overall fitness.

One Extreme Example In The Headlines

The study that made some of the biggest headlines to date was a study out of McMaster University that appeared in the journal *PLOS ONE* in April 2016. This study by Gillen et al. (2016) suggested that 1-minute of high-intensity exercise may yield the same benefits as 45-

minutes of moderate exercise. They compared sprint interval training (SIT) to moderate-intensity continuous training (MICT) using sedentary men as their test subjects. The SIT group did three workout sessions per week consisting of three 20 second "all-out" cycle sprints (~500W) separated by two minutes of much easier cycling (50W). The MICT group did 45-minutes of cycling at ~70% of their maximum heart rate (~110W) (Abstract – Methods section, para. 1).

At the end of twelve weeks, Gillen et al. (2016) concluded that:
"... a SIT protocol involving 3 minutes of intense intermittent exercise per week, within a total time commitment of 30 minutes, is as effective as 150 minutes per week of moderate-intensity continuous training for increasing insulin sensitivity, cardiorespiratory fitness and skeletal muscle mitochondrial content in previously inactive men" (Conclusion section, para. 1)

What This Means To Us
You need to train for speed and stamina. This study, and others like it, suggest that we may gain by doing both at once. That interests me because your cardiovascular training can add to your speed training time.

My HIIT Routine
Most of the studies on HIIT, that I've read, have incorporated either sprinting or use of a stationary bike. I don't believe that either of those types of workouts translate well to martial arts. I believe that, when working on stamina, you should work the muscle groups that will be put into action during actual performance.

Never in my life will I allow my HIIT routine to be videoed or photographed. That's because the laughing would never end. You're just going to have to use your imagination. My kicks all start with a fast chamber with the knee raised as fast as possible. I also use a lot of strikes that enlist the use of my shoulders and arms. For me, a perfect high-intensity workout would incorporate fast leg lifts, like running in place with high knees, and punches like, well, punches. So, during the high-intensity segments, I run in-place and use a punching motion at the same time as fast and hard as I possibly can.

Many times in this book, I've encouraged you to use visualization. Maybe, in this case, you can give me a break and skip it.

Joking aside, I believe this to be a perfect HIIT routine for martial arts. It utilizes relevant movements, works pertinent muscle groups, engages large muscle groups, and permits maximum speed. Your body type or martial art style may lead you to a different routine. Just ensure that you are actually doing HIIT, so that you reap full benefits.

Making It Happen

My HIIT routine consists of a 2-minute warmup followed by six to eight 30-second high-intensity segments that are separated by 2-minute segments of moderate activity. I finish the workout with a 3-minute cooldown at moderate activity level. I push each 30-second segment to my absolute max. I have to tell you that every time that I do this routine I spend a lot of the workout wondering if I'm gambling with my 57-year-old ticker. It's that intense.

If you choose to try HIIT, as with any speed workout, protect your joints. Don't fully extend your arms and run on a cushioned surface.

A HIIT Miss For Martial Artists

I don't recommend shadow sparring for the high-intensity segments of a HIIT routine. There is far too much rest even in intense shadow sparring. The high-intensity segments should be like sprinting or all-out cycling. The exertion is constant. Shadow sparring just doesn't fit the bill.

A Big Warning About HIIT

Along with the recent scientific evidence has come a massive herd of those who wish to capitalize on the masses who are more than willing to believe anything to get fit and lose weight by committing to only a few minutes of exercise. Be careful. There is a lot of hype, and there are a lot of wild health claims being thrown all over the Internet. If you choose to try a HIIT routine, ensure that you are learning from a reputable source. Also, data is still coming in. Stay informed to ensure that you are doing the safest and most effective routine possible.

Shadow Sparring

While I don't recommend shadow sparring for HIIT, I do recommend it for speed training. Many high-profile boxing coaches consider shadow sparring to be the best speed training exercise. Shadow sparring has many benefits. You can work on balance, technique, strategy, accuracy, efficiency, and speed at the same time. You can also experiment with no concern about defending yourself as you would in actual sparring. While shadow sparring is a great speed workout, it is not a substitute for actual sparring. You still need to spend as much time as possible sparring a skilled training partner.

Making It Happen

Always visualize an opponent when shadow sparring. Throw every technique with purpose and with a target in mind. Proper form is as important during shadow sparring as it is at any other time. You're not just working out; you're developing skills and habits too. Don't spend a single moment practicing a bad habit.

When you shadow spar, take the intensity up a notch. No matter how much you try, shadow sparring never matches the intensity of facing an actual opponent. Be careful though to protect your body during intense shadow sparring. Uncontrolled movements or overextending can easily cause injury.

Training When You Are Tired

You don't perform as well or learn as well when you are fatigued. That's another reason I don't like to combine conditioning and skills training.

When you are fatigued, you lose mental focus and your form suffers. Do this often, and you can develop some seriously bad habits.

I'm sure some of you are balking right now because I obviously don't understand the value of learning perseverance, heart, chi, etc. through the struggle of having to dig deep within one's self to triumph over one's own limits. Sure, I do. So, I'll clarify. The kind of training that forces you to dig deep and demand more of yourself than you thought possible is absolutely essential to martial art training. And, there is some conditioning benefit to that kind of training. The problem is that you just can't do this kind of training consistently enough to qualify as a good conditioning regimen. It is just too taxing and should be reserved for times when the student is ready to take their art to a new higher level.

Earlier, I said that conditioning and skills training should not be combined. This is primarily true when learning new skills or when skills have not been perfected. During those periods, you must train with proper form to ensure that what makes it to subconscious proficiency is correct. Once you reach that point, everything changes. Once you can perform with full subconscious proficiency, the next step is to learn to perform those skills under more and more demanding conditions. This is how you become both tough and skilled, but proper skill must come first. While pushing through fatigue, you must still ensure that you don't develop poor habits by continually using poor form.

This is why in the description of my HIIT routine above, I said that I use a "punching motion." I would never train actual technique when my goal is to push myself into extreme fatigue.

An Exercise To Increase Your Kicking Speed

In Chapter 14, I make the case for using a single kicking chamber for nearly all of your kicks. My chamber brings my knee straight up much like when doing a knee lift. Yours may be very different. Regardless,

Strength and Conditioning

the speed of your kicks is extremely dependent on executing the chamber very fast. Working the chamber without fully executing the kick is an effective way to train kicking speed. You should be chambering a minimum of one hundred times per leg per workout. If you are doing very few fully executed kicks, you may need to add many more reps. This exercise doesn't replace training fully executed kicks. It is only meant to augment your kick training. This is also a great way to help maintain kicking speed during times that you need to reduce stress on your knees or hip joints.

Making It Happen

Chamber high and chamber *FAST*. Make every rep explosive as if kicking at maximum speed. Keep your hands up the entire time and maintain your fighting stance the entire time. You're conditioning the muscles involved in most of your kicks and contributing to the motor engrams (for kicking) that you learned about in Chapter 4. If necessary, to maintain proper form, reset between reps. You're training the speed of the chamber, not how quickly you can complete the set of reps.

Generally Speaking Of Conditioning For Speed

I believe that speed workouts should be designed to be very similar to how you plan to perform. Workout in the same stance and with similar motion. The differences that make it a workout are the intensity, repetition, and the level of protection that you employ. If you're working on kicking speed and power, you need to put in time either working the components of the kick, like fast leg lifts to chamber while in the kicking stance, or working the kick itself. In an actual fight, you might throw that kick with reckless abandon. That can easily end with an injury that may well be worth it if the kick saves your life. When training though, your goal is improvement of conditioning and form. The last thing that you want to do is rack up an injury. So, keep your training incrementally more demanding, but also keep it safe so that you can perform when it's time.

9

Flexibility
Get your foot off the brake.

FLEXIBILITY, AND HOW YOU PURSUE IT, HAS A massive impact on your speed. Yeah, I said massive. I know, we don't typically think of flexibility when we think of speed, but we should. A flexible body moves freely and easily. That's faster, much faster. Trying to perform with an inflexible body is like trying to drive a car with one foot on the brake as your inflexibility restrains your movement. If you're like most martial artists, you work hard to increase your flexibility. Unfortunately though, your stretching routine is probably sabotaging your speed and even your flexibility. There is a lot more to flexibility than sitting on the floor straining to do a split.

Flexibility Is Not Just For High Kickers

Flexibility is important to your speed even if you are not a high kicker. Muscle tension will slow your movement. Even if you learn to relax your muscles, tension will remain if you lack flexibility. A lack of flexibility can not only slow your physical movement, it can also be devastating to your balance and stamina, which in turn will reduce your speed and effectiveness.

You're Probably Making A Huge Mistake

If you do any static stretching before your workout, you're doing more harm than good. This is a BIG deal. That's why I'm going to repeat it throughout this chapter. Static stretching fatigues your muscles. It reduces your explosiveness, and it increases injuries. The good news is that the fix is very easy, and the gains from the fix are nearly immediate. Never static stretch first, never. We'll get into the details shortly.

So How Does A Lack Of Flexibility Slow Me Down?

The first thing you need to understand is what is going on in your body when it moves. During most limb movements, there is a muscle, or group of muscles, that contract in order to move a part of your body. Those muscles are termed the agonist or agonists. There are also muscles that have the potential to slow or stop your movement, or even move you in the opposite direction. These are termed the antagonistic muscles. Some of these groups of muscles are called antagonistic pairs.

Very simply stated, antagonistic muscles are the muscles that would be put into action to move you in the opposite direction that you are attempting to move. A good example is the relationship of the biceps and the triceps. To retract your arm, as if to bring a drink to your mouth, your biceps would contract and pull your forearm close to your upper arm. In this case, the biceps would be the agonists. Your triceps must relax to allow your forearm to move because if they were to contract, they would cause your arm to extend. Therefore, the triceps, in this case, are the antagonists. If your goal was to extend your arm as if to point to a distant object, the two muscle groups would trade roles with the triceps being the agonists, and the biceps being the antagonists.

The antagonistic muscles serve a very vital role in your movement. Their tension in opposition to your movement serves to stabilize your body. Additionally, they control deceleration, and therefore, speed. You can quickly see that any unneeded tension in the antagonistic muscles will impede your movement because those muscles will be working in opposition to your desired movement. It would be much like trying to drive your car forward with one foot on the accelerator and one foot on the brake. Get your foot off the brake.

Your Brain Knows Where You Are

Your brain knows where all of your body parts are at all times. This is called proprioception. Proprioception is what enables you to touch your nose with your eyes closed. It is also one way that your brain attempts to protect your muscles from injury. Your brain knows where your range of motion limits are, and it knows when you approach those limits. When you are approaching those limits, tension is created in the antagonistic muscles by contracting them to slow or stop your movement in an effort to prevent you from exceeding that limit. If that limit is short of the point you are attempting to move to, the result will be slowed or even stopped motion. If you are moving with enough intensity, the result will include torn muscles and/or connective tissues. To be fast, your antagonistic muscles must be relaxed to prevent slowing of your intended motion. Flexibility extends the range of motion that you can utilize at full speed.

Unless You Like Throwing Yourself To The Floor...

Kicking beyond your comfortable range of flexibility can adversely affect your balance. Recovering from a loss of balance requires time. That loss of time reduces your speed. Even worse, you may land on the floor.

When a kick reaches the limit of your range of flexibility, it will be stopped by the antagonistic muscles. If the kicking leg is still engaged in substantial motion at this point its inertia must be absorbed in some manner. Either the antagonistic muscles and/or associated tendons will absorb the energy, which may tear them, or the support leg will be dragged out of position. In the worst scenario, both will occur.

When the support leg is dragged out of position, you will, to some degree, be forced off balance. You may even find yourself on the floor.

Recovery from any degree of loss of balance makes you vulnerable to attack and requires substantial time for recovery. Any time consumed for anything other than your defense or attack is a reduction in your speed. To be fast, always work within your comfortable range of motion. To better utilize your abilities, extend your comfortable range of motion by becoming more flexible.

You Are Stretching Wrong!

Most martial art classes start with students sitting on the floor doing static stretching. The instructor will tell you to, "hold that stretch." Often the stretches are held for thirty seconds or more. Some instructors will even walk around the room and push down on their students' backs to force them further into the stretch. Some instructors will tell their students to push to the point of pain or even to push through pain. Then, they will tell their students that stretching prevents injuries. They're doing what they've always done and they're doing it because it is what their instructor was taught and has always done. It is wrong and it is killing your speed.

Static stretching is fatiguing to the muscles and should never be performed before a dynamic activity. Period. The medical community now believes that static stretching reduces explosiveness and speed. Most recent studies also indicate that static stretching not only does not reduce injuries, it actually increases injuries. Did you get that? It can increase injuries. If you push to the point of pain, you may not even need to wait for the injury. You could easily have damaged your muscles and/or tendons already. Most often the damage is minor, but it can have big consequences. In the short term, you will reduce your speed and explosiveness. In the long term, you may do serious damage to your muscles and tendons. You may also be setting yourself up for a serious injury when training or performing.

Fatiguing and/or damaging your muscles and tendons before any dynamic activity is detrimental to your performance and speed.

Just Never

By sitting on the floor straining for that split before class, you have fatigued your muscles, and you have quite likely damaged them. That's right. You have reduced your explosiveness, and you have increased your risk of injury. Great. Now, let's all get up and expect to be able to perform with speed and power. This is senseless and needs to stop.

- **NEVER** stretch without proper and adequate warm-up. Break a sweat and fully warm your muscles before taxing them.
- **NEVER** engage in static stretching before training, competition, or any time that you plan to perform soon afterward. Think about it. How much sense does it make to tear down and fatigue your muscles before using them? Isometric and proprioceptive neuromuscular facilitation (PNF) stretches are even worse because they intentionally cause muscle fatigue. If done properly, the fatigue can be intense. **Save all of these types of stretches for your post workout and cool-down stretches.**
- **NEVER** stretch to the point of pain. Stretching to the point of pain can be damaging to muscles and tendons and should never be done, period. How did anyone ever think that this was a good idea?
- **NEVER** do ballistic stretches. **Never.** This is another stretch that can injure and injure quickly. Ballistic stretches are stretches that involve fast, uncontrolled motions that can easily exceed your present range of motion causing potentially severe injury.
- **NEVER** allow a partner to push or pull you to the point of pain or beyond. Leave that type of stretching to the movies. Nothing good happens during this type of stretching. If you have an instructor who insists on pushing on your back to force you down while stretching, leave. That's right. Leave. You don't need to be there. Find a competent instructor.
- **NEVER** strain when stretching. Regardless of the type of stretching, you must relax when attempting to increase your range. If the antagonistic muscles are fighting against the stretch,

Flexibility

they and the associated connective tissue can easily be damaged. Always consciously relax the muscles you are stretching as much as possible during the stretch. This goes for the stretching portion of isometric and PNF stretches as well.
- **NEVER** stretch an injured area until medically cleared to do so. Stretching injured muscles and tendons can greatly increase the damage and recovery time.

Do This Instead

Dynamic stretching utilizes motion within your static-passive range of flexibility. Dynamic stretching has a long list of benefits that translate directly to greater speed. Dynamic stretching requires only a few reps to be fully effective. Once you have stretched fully, you will typically maintain your full range of motion for at least the remainder of the day. You can stretch early and still perform with your full range of motion much later. Unlike other types of stretching, such as static, PNF (proprioceptive neuromuscular facilitation), and isometric, dynamic stretching does not fatigue or tear down the muscles. Dynamic stretching fits perfectly into the end of your warm-up (after your body is fully warmed up).

Dynamic stretching will prepare you to perform utilizing your full range of motion with no adverse effects on your explosiveness or stamina. It is the antagonists that we need to stretch. Those are the muscles that have the potential to slow or stop your movement. Static, PNF, and isometric stretches stress the antagonists, in some cases severely. Conversely, dynamic stretches work to reset your neurologic motion limits to their maximum with gentle movement that is compatible with how you plan to perform.

The routine below works just as well for the abductors. I strongly recommend holding onto something stable for support when dynamically stretching the abductors.

Save static, isometric, and PNF stretches for your cool-down period.

Making It Happen

This is the simple method that I use for stretching my hamstrings. Using this method, I can reach my full range of motion after just ten reps. That is extremely fast compared to static stretching. This is my routine. Your needs may be very different.

Do not attempt dynamic stretching without proper instruction.

1. Begin only after an adequate full-body warm-up.
2. Stand in a relaxed fighting stance. Holding something stable with one hand for support is recommended for safety.
3. Throughout the exercise consciously relax the leg that is going to be stretched.
4. Gently swing your leg forward and upward without bending the knee. Because the swing is gentle, you will need to use a little muscular effort to lift the leg in the final few inches.
5. That muscular lift at the end of the swing is important. Use it to gently muscle your leg up just a little higher with each swing.
6. Stop slightly before you reach your full range of motion. Do not let the leg travel to the point of causing pain. Always keep the swing entirely under control.
7. **NEVER** swing your leg without control in a ballistic motion. This can cause serious injury.
8. Repeat this exercise ten to twelve times for each leg. On each repetition, you will be able to swing slightly higher than the last. Let the lifting muscles do the work at the end of the swing. Never let the momentum of the swing force you higher.
9. When you become accustomed to this type of stretching, you should be able to reach your full range in a single set of ten to twelve repetitions.
10. With repeated use of dynamic stretching, you can easily increase your range of motion by gently increasing the travel of the swing by enlisting the lifting muscles increasingly as you reach the limit of your comfortable range of motion.

10

Mentally Fast

Get this wrong and nothing else will matter.

I REMEMBER THE FIRST TIME THAT I WALKED AWAY from a match and had to ask what I had done. My conscious mind had no recollection of the entire match. I was a little confused at first. This was just a short time after I had started studying the abilities of the mind, so it wasn't long until I realized that I had simply engaged the training that had been deeply placed in my subconscious mind. My conscious mind had gotten completely out of the way. I had dominated my opponent having never even had a point scored on me. Right then I knew this was a key to being extremely fast. Next, I started wondering why I had never been taught anything about how to elicit that level of performance before.

Speed is as at least as much mental as it is physical, probably even more so. Speed happens in the mind first. It is even easier for speed to die in the mind. Then, there is the mind's power to inflict adverse effects on your opponent's speed. Development of dominating speed demands that you understand and utilize the power that your mind can wield.

The human mind is much more powerful than you probably realize. At the time of this writing, I've spent thirty-six years studying the mind, learning ability, and intelligence. I teach people how to learn very fast, high-level problem solving, and how to be intelligent. The most interesting part is that the power was within them all along. It is within you as well. It's just a matter of using the brain as it was designed to be used.

Number One Rule Of Speed

For speed, rule number one is to keep your conscious mind out of the way. You're probably tired of hearing that by now, but this is so important that it's worth repeating. Conscious thought is slow. Training is all about moving skills to the subconscious mind, which is extremely fast. Train well, and then rely on your training.

If you must consciously think about a technique or skill, you haven't trained well enough to be fast. Period.

Believe, Whether You Believe Or Not

Belief is extremely powerful. Elite athletes in every sport actively use belief to push themselves to heights others can barely comprehend. For most people, the power of belief remains largely untapped.

I'm not talking about meaningless affirmations and touchy-feely-nonsensical-you-can-be-anything mantra chanting. I'm referring to the application of sound psychological principals. Unfortunately, most of you reading this will never so much as scratch the surface of your mind's power. That may sound a little negative, but it is fact. Countless books have been written on the power of belief that give you everything you need to put it into action. From the religious perspective of belief as faith in the Bible two thousand years ago to countless secular self-help titles written in modern times, belief is at the center of success. Still with all of this information available, only a few will embrace the concept.

Whether you believe it or not, what you believe is what you will become. Believe that you are fast, and you will become fast. Believe you are slow, and slow you will be. This may sound a little strange if you are not familiar with the psychology of belief, but it is fact. Just go with it. It works.

I know that at age 57 I'm still fast in large part because I believe that I am. I don't buy into the general belief that at my age I should be slowing down. I'm not a lemming. I control my reality. Kick everybody else out of your head and believe what serves you, not what you've always been told. Most of what people believe is based in that old adage that misery loves company. Let the miserable be miserable alone.

Train In Your Brain

Vividly imagining a physical activity fires the same neural pathways as actually engaging in the physical activity. That means vivid training in your brain pays dividends in reality. I had been doing this for many years when I first saw an elite athlete do this. It was an Olympic figure skater. The skater was sitting on the floor going over an upcoming routine with eyes closed. The skater's body executed abbreviated movements along with the imagined moves being executed fully in his mind's eye. Olympic athletes don't make a habit of wasting their time and effort. This skater knew that imagined training would contribute to better physical performance. These days you can see nearly all of the freestyle skiers and snowboarders at the top of the mountain doing the same thing.

This is an excellent way to train when you don't have the space or time to physically train. It's also a great way to experiment without physical risk. It saves wear on your joints and allows training when you are injured or too sore for a physical workout.

More importantly, this is a great place to build belief in your speed. You can be as fast as you want to be in your mind. There are no limits. I suggest though that you keep it in the realm of possibility, or you will risk having no positive impact on your belief.

Making It Happen

Just do what you do, but do it in your mind. Sit quietly and imagine. No meditation, chanting, or lotus position needed. It is important that the images be as vivid and realistic as possible. Include all of your senses that you can. The images can be from your perspective or from a third-person perspective. Just ensure that your technique is precise.

Some people have difficulty creating imagery in their mind. It is not necessary for you to see vivid images as long as you are imagining the movements as realistically as possible. The only big mistake that you can make is to think in words. Thinking in words happens primarily in your conscious mind. That's not where you need to be. Just daydream like you would daydream about anything else. If you are imagining the actions and the outcomes, you are effective.

This may not be easy in the beginning. If you have trouble or lose your image momentarily, simply take a breath and start again. Don't give up. Play until you win.

Powerful Focus

Mental focus is essential for success. You must first understand what focus is for a martial artist. Focus is exclusion of thought rather than intense thought. Focusing means applying yourself fully to the task at hand to the exclusion of all else. It does not mean intense concentration or fixation on a single aspect of the act or even the act itself. Intense concentration and fixation are products of mind consuming conscious thought. When fully focused on a fight, the martial artist has turned off all conscious thought and has given his or her body over to the subconscious mind, and the training that has been stored there. In this state, you are doing what you are doing and nothing else. You are as mentally fast as you will ever be, which means you can be as physically fast as you will ever be. When you finish the fight, you will most likely have to ask someone what you did. You will not be consciously aware at that time. It will most likely come to you later though.

A runner looking over his or her shoulder cannot run as fast as a runner who is focused on running to the exclusion of everything else. Any time spent thinking about something that you shouldn't be is time lost. That lost time means you either lost speed or gave speed to your opponent.

Making It Happen

Do not attempt this while doing anything that is even the slightest bit demanding of your attention for safety.

Force yourself to focus. That doesn't mean just when training. Make focus a habit; make it a normal part of you. If you don't already have a long attention span, this will not be easy at first.

Pick a specific task to focus on. It can be anything from cooking dinner to an educational assignment. Just don't select something that requires interaction with someone else. Select something that takes long enough to push the limits of your current ability to focus. Attempt to complete the task with zero thought of anything else. Single-minded execution is your goal. Do not think in words. Execute only. This may seem strange at first, but try until the light goes on. Trust me when you feel it you will know it. This will only be learned by doing. It will only be understood by experiencing. Turn those words off. I mean it! **DO NOT THINK IN WORDS!** Just do.

Your mind may wander soon after you start. Every time your mind wanders force it back on topic. When your mind wanders again, force it back again. Do not relent. Play until you win. Quitting is not an option. This is going to be frustrating, but the payoff is extremely powerful. As you progress, pick a task that takes longer.

Once you have command of your focus for three to five minutes, put it to work in sparring. To do this, explain to your sparring partner what you are doing or at least instruct your partner to keep contact light and controlled. Any time you are working on something new, you are at risk of injury due to distraction or disorientation. Always ensure that you've set yourself up to advance safely. Also, having to protect yourself will itself distract you from focusing.

When you are comfortable and feel functional enough, begin to put your new focus level into action in your full complement of training, sparring and fighting situations. When you are totally focused, totally engaged, you can use all of the speed that your body is physically capable of. Mental slowness will not exist.

The Popular Way To NEVER Train Focus

Focus for martial artists does not mean intense concentration on a single thought or subject. That is why common focus exercises are not only ineffective; they're detrimental. Typically, an instructor will tell the student to look at a spot on a wall and try to not look away for a minute, two minutes, or maybe longer. The goal is for the student to learn discipline and control in order to focus single-mindedly, rather than being subject to distractions from their surroundings as well as those within them in the form of distracting thoughts. This exercise has some seriously detrimental effects. Staring at the small spot narrows the student's field of view. That narrowing is primarily a mental function, but there is a physical component as well. Physically staring at the dot requires convergence of the student's eyes. That convergence further narrows the field of view.

More importantly, the student's mind is being trained to focus on a small area to the exclusion of its surroundings. Your mind is extremely adept at filtering and limiting your awareness. That is how you can be in a loud, crowded room and still hear an individual. Your mind filters out what is undesired. Vision is no different. The dot exercise is perfect for training to narrow your mental awareness. That combined with the convergence of your eyes is a perfect recipe for seriously narrowing your field of view. Develop that habit well, and you won't see 90% of your opponent's attacks coming.

Widen Your Field Of View

Do not do this when doing anything that demands your attention to ensure your safety.

You have more control over your field of view than you may realize. Unknowingly though, we often narrow our field of view. Control of your field of view can greatly increase your ability to respond to attacks and to take advantage of openings. Both of which contribute to increased speed.

Right now, without looking away from these written words, without moving your eyes at all, try to see/become aware of your surroundings to your left and right. If you are like most people, this required a little conscious effort. Typically, we tune those things out. All of those things you are now "seeing" were there all along and were being detected by your eyes. You had just tuned them out by narrowing your field of view mentally.

Long ago, I read about a basketball great, whose name I've long forgotten, who credited his ability to drive to the net to training himself to have a wider field of view. This wider view enabled him to be more aware of the threats and options that lay before him and around him.

Be aware that things in your peripheral vision will be slightly out of focus. That is just a result of how your eyes are designed. Begin to widen your field of view. This does not mean dart your eyes left and right. This is a mental function. In your mind, become aware of your full field of view.

Emotion

Keep emotion out of your training, sparring, and self-defense except to the extent that it is a motivating. Anger, fear, anxiety, and any other negative emotion can destroy your speed as well as your ability to execute skills that you otherwise would find to be easy. Fear and anger will cause rigidity and hesitation. Rigidity is slow. Hesitation is literally death to speed. Even otherwise positive emotions can be problematic. Being overly relaxed, confident, or anxious (ready to go) can be just as debilitating as fear and anxiety.

Don't confuse anger and motivation. Most beginners think that they are better, faster fighters when they are angry. They're wrong. You are a better fighter when you are calm, calculated, and executing your training systematically. You must be relaxed and clear-headed to be fast and effective. Be angry later, worry later, celebrate later, and feel pain later. Right now, it's all business. Do what you are doing. Period.

So, How Do I Turn Off Emotion?

Decide to. That sure sounds simplistic, but that is a first and most crucial step. Most people wouldn't know a real decision if it hit them in the face. Mostly they want, wish, and hope and that's only if it doesn't require work or commitment. They think that doing something like controlling their emotions is extremely difficult because that is what they have always been led to believe. If you are a mentally healthy person, that is far from the truth. Making a true decision based on a compelling reason is all powerful in the human mind. Decide that you will train and compete with a mind that is motivated by your goals rather than controlled by your emotions.

You may be thinking, "but emotion drives me," or "emotions are what make me human." Emotions are not absent from this process. Turning off emotion and thought doesn't mean that your mind is vacant. You still need to be operating with purpose, and purpose is derived from emotion. You want to win a match because of the emotions connected with winning. You want to execute effective self-defense because you want to avoid the negative emotions that come with being a victim. Emotion gives you purpose. Purpose fuels goals. Use those goals to create a mindset with which to operate. Your mindset is the state of mind that you choose to assume in order to accomplish your goal. That mindset is what you need to establish as your method of operation.

Making It Happen

Imagery is extremely powerful in the human mind. Imagine being a machine. Assume the role of that machine. Without emotion, it carries out its duties. Notice that I said, "without emotion" not without purpose. It continues regardless of what is going on around it. You can shoot at it, beat it, and set it on fire. Still, until incapacitated, it will relentlessly continue toward its goal. As someone who may need to use your fighting skills to defend yourself or others, you need this ability to single-mindedly get the job done. This is just as important when competing.

Is that a little confusing? Read the next section, "Is There A Nurse In The House?" You'll get the point.

Is There A Nurse In The House?

How about an analogy? I know a lady who is an emergency room nurse. One afternoon her young son had an accident at home that resulted in a very serious cut. He was bleeding profusely and needed medical attention ASAP. How lucky could he be? There was an ER nurse right there with him. Or, was there? The mother was terrified. She went into hysterics to the point of being immobilized. All of her training, knowledge, and experience as an ER nurse were nonexistent. No, there was not an ER nurse in the house. She was useless and actually impeded assistance from the boy's father who had to struggle to keep her out of the way. As callous as it may sound, she needed to turn off all emotion and get the job done as efficiently as possible by applying her expertise.

First responders, military personnel, doctors, and many others do this every day. In situations that would put most of us in the fetal position, they methodically get the job done. It's called relying on your training and working with purpose. It can be done, and it is not callous at all. It is peak efficiency. You can worry and be upset later. You can be frustrated and angry later. Give yourself maximum opportunity to win by training yourself to turn off all emotion. Be a machine.

The emergency room nurse could have taken on the purpose of rendering aid like a machine. She could have assumed the mindset of a skilled nurse and temporarily turned off the emotions of a mother in distress. Given the motivation of her purpose (to save her child) and the training committed to her subconscious mind, she could have functioned extremely efficiently and effectively at maximum speed. She would not have been operating mindlessly. She would just have pushed disabling emotion and conscious thought out of the way. After it was all over, she could cry, scream, and be angry if she wanted to, but only after her goal was accomplished as effectively as possible.

Making It Happen

For you, this means putting past failures, concerns about your training, fear, anxiety, self-doubt, pain, ego, disdain for your opponent, and anything else that is not mission oriented out of your mind. Think you can't do that? Make a decision and take on the mindset of getting the job done and executing your training. Any reward that will bring can serve as your motivation. From that point forward, it's all business. If you were running a race, you would run. You would do nothing else. You would think of nothing else. You would just run as fast and as effectively as possible. You would NEVER look over your shoulder for even a moment. Just get the job done. Well, you could worry about your next race, or that competitor that dissed you, or your sore toe, and just go ahead and lose. That's always an option. I think you get the point.

Relax

It's called tension for a reason. Being tense is tight. Tight is slow because tension resists movement. The tension that makes you tight starts in your mind. Even in self-defense situations, stay relaxed. Accomplish what needs to be done. You can worry and be tense later. Give yourself every possibility to win. One of the best ways to relax is to know what you are doing. Train effectively and work within your own limits.

What Did I Do?

You'll know that you've got the mental game right when you finish a match or sparring session and are unable to remember what you did. Conscious thought played no part. It was all subconscious execution of deep training with words, debate, and emotion absent. However, if you can't remember what you did and you got stomped, it may be time to reassess your training.

Conditioning Matters Mentally

We know that conscious thought is slow. We know that focus is fast. The best possible way to lose focus and start thinking is to be tired in a fight. When you are tired, you think and not about winning. You think about surviving. Unless you get lucky, you will lose. You will definitely be slow. The only possible way to turn this situation around is to reach deep down inside, turn every single conscious thought off, and explode into a mass of action based solely on your training with extreme speed and efficiency. Or, you could have conditioned properly and never gotten tired in the first place. It is a mental game, but conditioning matters.

Getting Into Your Opponent's Head

We know that anger, frustration, fear, and conscious thought will make us slower. It will do the same for your opponent. Any time you can mess with your opponent's mental game, do so. Some people are more easily influenced than others, but everyone is vulnerable.

Even highly trained professional fighters are vulnerable. Calling an opponent out even before the matchup is finalized, trash talking, the stare-down at the weigh-in, refusing to shake hands at the start of the match, taunting during the match, etc. are all about getting into the opponent's head. Some of it smacks of poor sportsmanship and most of it does not fit into the strict honor code of some traditional martial arts, but it is none the less effective. What you do is up to you. It's all about what you are willing to do to win.

Enjoy Getting Hit

That's right. Enjoy getting hit even though you hate it. Even how you react to getting hit can have an effect on your speed. It's not natural to not be bothered by being hit. It's natural to be upset, scared, and angered. Those emotions will cause tension and an adrenaline dump. Both will destroy your speed. Decide to deal with it. You're learning to fight after all (or you're a fighter already). Other people have done it. So can you.

When I was a teenager, I saw an old western movie. A guide was helping a wagon train of settlers that was heading west. In one scene, they were high in the Rocky Mountains when one of the settlers fell over a cliff. He screamed all the way down. Indians heard the screams, so they knew right where to find and attack the settlers. When the attack was over, the guide chewed out everybody and told them that the guy was going to die anyway, so he should have stayed quiet to protect everyone else. Later in the movie, two more settlers fell over a cliff. You saw them falling through the air for a hundred feet or so, but they were completely silent. They didn't give in to emotion. They sucked it up and did what they had to no matter how hard it was. That lesson has stayed with me ever since, and it should stay with you too.

Don't believe that it is difficult to overcome fear. You control you. Don't believe that anything else controls you. Do what needs to be done. It's all business.

11

Accuracy and Timing

Missing is speed lost.

Accuracy and timing are two more topics that rarely come up in discussions of speed. Being fast and accurate makes you dangerous. Accuracy requires timing as well as navigation. Getting to the wrong place fast doesn't meet the definition of speed for martial artists. Time elapses until effective completion. Nothing good happens if you miss your target whether it's a strike, a block, or a takedown. When you get to your target accurately, you've made your way to effective completion. If you miss your target, speed for that technique, in terms of effective completion, is at zero. The same is true if you arrive early or late. In terms of time, the clock never stopped because effective completion never occurred. At that point, speed becomes all about recovery or redirection in order to effectively complete another attack or defense.

Accuracy Is Four Dimensional

When most people think of accuracy, they think of hitting a target as measured on the vertical axis and the horizontal axis. For the martial artist, accuracy is much more than that. Yes, the martial artist must connect with a target, which involves pinpointing a strike or block on the vertical and horizontal. The martial artist must also accurately deliver power at the correct distance and time. This requires all aspects of the technique to complete at just the right place as well as at the right moment and distance. For a punch, that means everything from the feet through the hips to the shoulder to the extension of the arm to the final movement of the fist must happen at the correct moment, at the correct distance, at the correct force, and at the correct place in order to expend power into the target at the desired level. All of this must be coordinated with a moving target that has a mind of its own and that doesn't want to be hit.

To be fast, you must be loose until the instant that your power is to be delivered to your target. To transfer power into your target, the muscles involved must be fully tensed at the moment of impact. Expending your power too early or too late will make the technique as inaccurate as being off vertically or horizontally.

> **The Definition Of Speed For Martial Artists**
> *"The time that elapses from perception to effective completion."*

You're Built For This

There you have the four dimensions: vertical, horizontal, distance, and time. There is a tremendous amount of calculation and physics involved in all of that. At a glance, this all sounds nearly impossible. Actually, our bodies and brains are well prepared for this kind of targeting. It is something that we already do routinely. In fact, nearly every movement you make involves a degree of targeting. It's not just us higher brained humans who can pull this off. How do you think your dog manages to catch a ball? There are regions of the brain that work in concert with your binocular vision (two eyes with fields of view that overlap) for targeting. The thought processes there operate independently of conscious thought, so the task is accomplished extremely fast, nearly instantly.

Most of the targeting that you do routinely are functions that you've done since you were very young. The behaviors are a natural part of your existence because you've practiced them many thousands of times. Not to mention that you started small and advanced as the years passed. If you played sports from a very young age, such as baseball, football, or soccer, your targeting in those sports is probably much better than an adult who is just starting in one of those sports. This is especially true the younger you started because the young brain learns more efficiently than the adult brain (the brain architecture is actually different).

If you started your martial arts studies at a very early age, you have a tremendous advantage in targeting because, if trained properly, effective targeting has become a natural part of what you do. This is your goal now, no matter if you are just starting or if you've studied for decades. Make it a natural part of you.

The Big Secret Is To Actually Try

The typical martial art student thinks mostly about volume rather than accuracy. Sparring usually turns into a kick and punch festival. There is little consideration about where the techniques are going, but there sure are plenty of them. There are two reasons for this. One is that they often aren't given finite objectives for targeting and timing. The other is that classroom sparring often takes on a workout feel rather than that of a fight. The students just plain never get into a score or be scored on mindset. It's more aerobics than sparring.

You should be gearing up and sparring with contact (even if it's light) and purpose. With purpose means that if it doesn't need to be thrown, you don't throw it. If you do throw it, have a definite target. When you miss, learn from it. Reassess, adjust, and go again. This all applies to your defensive movement as well.

In your mind, every sparring session should be a match or a fight. Even if it's a no-contact session. Execute every strike with purpose and a definite target. It's best if your opponent knows what you're doing so you can include working through defenses. If your opponent chooses to do aerobics, continue on using them as a target. This doesn't mean that you pound them when they don't expect it. You can still stay within the confines of the rules.

Timing

There is no chapter dedicated to timing in this book. That doesn't mean it is not important. Timing is an integral part of speed. Rather than separate timing for discussion, I have included it in the discussions of many other subjects throughout this book. Timing is too intertwined with other skills to be separated. Yeah, other instructors will tell you to learn timing by training on a speed bag or double-ended speed bag. All those do is teach you how to hit a speed bag or a double-ended speed bag. You're way better off to invest your training time in sparring.

Timing your opponent is a skill that is gained only through experience and lots of it. It is also one of the first things to go when you take time off. Mastering the other elements in this book will make you very fast. Being fast gives you a greater margin for error in timing as you will be less likely to be late, and you will have more time to recover if you do mistime a technique.

The most important thing I can tell you about timing is to learn to take advantage of your speed by initiating your movement earlier. Instead of countering after your opponent completes a kick or strike begin your counter just as your opponent's technique gets out of the gate. Be mindful to block or evade as you counter. Try to score before your opponent's technique gets to you. This has a demoralizing effect on your opponent, which can lead to frustration, which leads to conscious thought, which slows everything for your opponent.

When To Initiate A Counter

Once you have developed very fast movement, you can begin to counter much earlier. Your counter should be executed at the instant the attacking strike or kick begins. That means when it has moved at most, two or three inches. If you read a telegraph, you can often execute the counter before the attack even begins. Countering at the moment your opponent begins an attack is very effective and will frustrate your opponent, which is always a speed win. It also makes it much more difficult for your opponent to reset or execute a follow-up technique. Countering this early requires fast movement, timing, and the ability to read your opponent.

Being a dominant counter fighter is extremely effective in sparring and tournament fighting. Not only does it adversely affect your opponent's mental game, it has a positive effect on the judges who I believe are quicker to award points to an obviously dominant competitor.

The Targeting Mindset

A little repetition for emphasis... Never just spar. Never just kick. Never just punch. Always have a target in mind and always try to improve your accuracy. Do everything that you do with the intent of perfect targeting. Your goal is to make accuracy as automatic as possible. It is not something that you turn on and off. Your goal is for accuracy to become a natural part of you.

Balance

Balance affects accuracy, and accuracy affects balance. To be accurate, you need to launch your movement from a predictable and stable body position. This is especially important when in motion. Dynamic balance is key to the body control that will set you up to accurately strike and block. See Chapter 5 for much more on balance.

Training

No matter what you're training or why, always have a target in mind. Even when striking and blocking nothing but thin air always aim your techniques. You may only be working on your conditioning, but you must still aim every technique. Never miss a chance to reinforce the always-on accuracy mindset that will eliminate the need for conscious thought. And, never settle for close enough.

Moving Targets

Have you ever noticed that most people don't like to get hit? They tend to block or move out of the way. Sometimes even both. The more skilled your opponent is, the more unpredictable and effective their movement will be. So, you must train your accuracy on randomly moving targets. Sparring is absolutely the best way to train your accuracy on unpredictably moving targets. You can also work with a partner using focus mitts or any type of handheld target that can be quickly moved. Training with focus mitts allows you to make more powerful contact than is advisable in sparring.

Making It Happen

Enlist the assistance of a skilled partner. Have your partner hold pads or targets appropriate for the techniques that you are training. In the beginning, have your partner move the target slow enough for you to connect a high percentage of attempts. Continue this level until you are connecting a high percentage. Then, your partner can begin to move the target quicker and more randomly. Over time progressively move up to a speed that mimics the movement of an actual opponent.

- In the beginning, use a larger target to increase safety.
- Keep the movement as realistic as possible.
- Hold the targets at a realistic height and position.
- The targets must be at realistic distances.

- Don't stare at the target. Aim your eyes where you normally aim them so that your training is relevant to actual performance.
- Ensure that your partner doesn't move the target right before impact. This can be dangerous for your joints.

Missing

Misses are inevitable especially when beginning accuracy training on randomly moving targets. Even at advanced levels, misses are going to happen. If you are not missing, you need to increase the difficulty level. If you're not missing in sparring, you need to be fighting more skilled opponents. Misses can be very frustrating as well. Strive for accuracy but mentally accept misses. Never allow misses to cause you to lose focus or control.

Protect Your Joints

Those misses are dangerous for your joints especially if the technique is fully extended with power. You must protect your body when training. Training is useless if your body is too damaged to perform when needed. Always strive to control your power and protect your body especially when trying something that is new for you.

Offensive Misses

Offensive misses are devastating to speed especially when striking with power. Misses, except for jabs and other harassment type strikes, typically require commitment of motion. A miss can leave you in a vulnerable position and often in your opponent's territory. Train to recover with the same speed with which you strike. Martial artists who strike with superior speed are few. Martial artists who recover with superior speed are downright rare. This is an easy way to gain a tremendous speed advantage. Train yourself to return your weapons to chamber instantly and in the most direct path possible. I can't stress this enough. A machine gun is effective because when it strikes, it instantly chambers another round and is ready to strike again. Never let a miss linger, drop, or otherwise take a lumbering, inefficient path back to chamber. This goes for feet as well as hands.

This all actually goes for hits as well. When anything leaves chamber, put it back into chamber immediately, so that it can be used again. Getting back to chamber is as much a technique as any strike. So, effective completion of the rechamber meets the definition of speed.

Defensive Misses

Defensive misses can be very serious. When a defensive technique misses, it typically means that something got through. The truth here is that you can't block everything. The important thing is to rechamber quickly to be ready to defend again or to launch a counterattack. Rechamber with the same speed that you strike and defend.

Training For Misses

It is not enough to just read how to handle misses. Put it into your training. No matter what accuracy training method you choose, it is imperative that you train for misses just as diligently as you train for accuracy. Apply everything that you learn about speed in this book to your recovery from misses and hits. Again, this cannot be stressed enough. There is a tremendous speed advantage that can be gained here.

Most Of You Never Learned Accuracy

In a typical martial art school, you will see most of the students sparring with flailing arms and legs that fly around with absolutely no purpose whatsoever. There is no accuracy because there isn't even a target in mind. When it comes time for breaking, the board holders leave with mangled fingers. That's because even if accuracy is taught, very few students actually train for accuracy. If you've now decided to pursue accuracy and speed, you must walk before you run.

Making It Happen
1. Go back to basic strikes and kicks on the heavy bag.
2. Pick a target on the bag. That can be an existing logo or

Accuracy and Timing

scratch, or you can stick a piece of tape on it.
3. Stand in a sparring/fighting stance.
4. Strike the target with your chosen technique.
5. Start slow and easy.
6. Keep your stance and movements as realistic as possible.
7. Add power and speed only when you begin to consistently hit your target. I mean every time with zero thought needed.
8. Once your foundation is built move on to more difficult targets. Don't overtrain skills that have no real application.

If this seems basic and rudimentary, that's because it is. Never underestimate the power of mastering the basics. Get on with it.

Training For Accuracy And Speed

Below is a list of the most common accuracy training tools. All of them can be effective. Sparring is still best, but sometimes you need supplemental training and training that allows for power strikes.

- **Heavy bag** – Good for beginners because it hangs stationary until impact and provides a large target. This is safer because misses can be damaging to joints. Due to its weight, it is good for practicing power as well. Its heavy weight prevents it from moving very far during hand strikes making it a good tool for beginners to train combinations.
- **Shield targets** – A large padded target that is held by a partner. Safer again because of its large target area. A shield can allow for slightly more realistic training because it can be moved randomly by your training partner.
- **Focus targets** – Small handheld padded targets. Most often used for kicks. They typically have a handle that positions the holder's hand several inches from the target area. They can easily be moved at random but rarely are in common practice.
- **Punch mitts** - Heavily padded gloves that are worn by a training partner. They can be easily moved. These can be effective tools if used properly. Unfortunately, most users hold them in very

impractical positions, and when they move them, they do so in predictable patterns.
- **Double end bag** – A small spherical bag that is attached at the top and bottom by elastic cords. When the bag is hit, it will rebound immediately and unpredictably. Because it moves erratically when struck, it provides a very challenging target for follow-up strikes. This is the go-to accuracy bag for boxers.

Form Before Fast

Learn proper form before adding a technique to your accuracy training. It's not unusual to see even long-time martial artists struggling to connect a single strike when sparring. Blocking is often worse. Not only have they not trained their targeting skills, they have not even learned to properly execute the techniques that they are throwing. If someone just wants to play karate, that's fine for them. If you want to be effective, or even exceptional, you must train and master proper form in your techniques. Only then can you execute with speed and accuracy. That means intense training with purpose.

Making It Happen

You should be training accuracy for every technique. Breadwinner techniques, the ones that you rely on the most, should receive even more attention and training.

Select a go-to technique to improve. Let's say you've selected the lead foot roundhouse kick. Dissect that kick. It doesn't matter if you've been throwing roundhouse kicks for ten years. Dissect it anyway. Understand proper form from the support foot up through the chamber to the hips to contact. Then, put that form into practice every day with conscious focused execution. Every practice kick should be thrown with all four dimensions of targeting in mind. Start out slowly, very slowly, with only a mental image of your target. Then, move to a heavy bag where distance targeting can be trained. Place a piece of tape on the heavy bag as a target and make every kick count. Then, progress to a focus target held by a partner. Train until proper form and execution are automatic. Finally, move to dynamic situations where the kick combines with body movement and strategy, such as in sparring. Have a partner hold a large shield while moving similarly to sparring. Once you are connecting a very high percentage, move on to practice sparring with a skilled training partner.

If you plan on using a setup technique for the kick that you are working on, incorporate that setup into your accuracy training very early on and continue all the way into sparring. Of course, you won't always use the setup, so practice with and without it.

Most Focus Mitt Drills Are Counterproductive

I say that because most often the mitts are held in a single position. The trainee strikes repeatedly in the exact same position. You can easily become very fast doing this. Unfortunately, you may have noticed that people move. Overtraining for a single position and distance will develop deeply rooted habits that you may find will limit your adaptability and timing. It's okay to keep those mitts, or any other target, stationary when you are in the early stages of training accuracy for a newly acquired technique, but get them moving as soon as you've gained proficiency. Your goal is effective speed and accuracy.

Accuracy And Timing Cannot Be Isolated

Efficiency, balance, distance, form, flexibility, power, and every other component of your martial art skillset are involved in accuracy and timing. When training, always incorporate as many of these components as possible by making your training mimic your performance goals as closely as you safely can.

Defensive Accuracy

Your defense needs to be as fast as your offense. Martial artists often neglect defensive accuracy. Practicing blocks is a common segment of nearly every class, but accuracy is largely left to chance. There is a common refrain of "keep your hands up," and sometimes there are some line drills that include blocking, but realistic, deliberate training of blocking accuracy is nearly nonexistent. This is another chance to do what others don't in order to rise above the crowd.

Making It Happen

Enlist the help of a skilled training partner. Gear up heavily and do some one-sided sparring. It's one-sided because you will be on defense only while your partner is on offense only. Foregoing offense allows you to focus on accuracy and timing of your blocks. Your partner should keep the attacks as realistic as possible, using the same tactics that would be employed in whatever type of performance that you are training for, be it competition, full-contact, or self-defense.

During the session, you should be working on timing your defenses in order to effect them as early in the attack as possible. Keep your mind clear and try to perceive and respond to the attack at the moment that it is initiated. You should find yourself firing your defenses before you even realize what you're doing. See Train It #1 (page 25) and #2 (page 32) in Chapter 3.

Ensure that your blocks are not only accurate but effective as well. Effective completion is just as important for defense as it is for offense. That means you must select a useful target. For example, blocking a ridge hand attack at the inside of the elbow can leave the entire forearm and hand an unimpeded path to your head.

This exercise is meant to allow you the freedom to develop your accuracy and timing skills without the added pressure of effecting your offense. This is just a stepping stone. Don't stay here. You will only perfect your accuracy and timing during actual sparring while engaging in offense as well as defense.

12

Telegraphing

Don't give your opponent advance notice.

TELEGRAPHING IS ANYTHING THAT SIGNALS TO your opponent what you are going to do before you do it. This reduces your opponent's perception time effectively increasing your delivery time. In other words, telegraphing gives your opponent advance notice that something is coming and provides additional time for your opponent to prepare and respond. You haven't lost speed. You've given it away.

> **I don't want my opponent to know I'm going to strike until shortly after impact.**

The most common telegraph is the wind-up. This is very common with beginning martial artists and is the one that you are most likely familiar with. It is the motion of pulling the fist backward before delivering it forward in an effort to strike with additional power. It is not uncommon for an experienced fighter to deliver a counter-strike before the novice even gets the punch halfway to its target. The windup is a glaring telegraph. There are many others, some of which are nearly imperceptible. Regardless of how tiny the telegraph is, the results are the same, reduced speed.

Wind Up Losing

The wind-up can be applied to nearly any technique, but here, we're going to look at a reverse punch. This also applies to a cross or straight punch. The wind-up happens when the fist is first drawn back before beginning its forward motion. As stated above, this is typically done in an effort to deliver more power. That's not always the case though. Many martial artists wind-up, however slightly, every strike and block they execute just because of poor form.

The first, and most important, problem with this is that it gives your opponent advance notice that the punch is coming. That alone is enough to negate the effectiveness of the punch. The second problem is that the wind-up adds to the distance that the fist must travel on its way to its target, which consumes time. The third problem is that the fist must decelerate and stop its rearward motion before beginning its acceleration forward.

It's easy to see that the wind-up can be devastating to your speed because the entire duration of the wind-up is time that is added to the delivery of the punch. To make matters worse, often the shoulder and upper torso will be shifted rearward as well. This adds even more time and distance as your center of gravity and body position must be stopped, reversed, and moved back to its original position before the punch can begin moving forward of its original position.

Making It NOT Happen

This isn't as easy as you might think. It's not as simple as stopping the wind-up motion. Most often when I convince someone to eliminate the wind-up motion, they begin to punch with just their arm and lose the ability to generate real power. That's fine if they're throwing a jab or a snapping technique. In the case of a power punch though, this is a serious problem. The root of the problem is that they don't understand proper power punching form. The student now must not only learn proper and effective punching form, they must also unlearn the poor and telegraphic form that is most likely a deep-rooted habit.

You must learn to execute your punches from chamber with only forward motion. You must fire the strike from exactly where your weapon is with no movement that isn't a part of the striking motion. For strikes with any power at all, this includes your legs, hips, torso, and shoulders which are all involved to varying degrees depending on the power you're delivering. For a full explanation of how to deliver a power punch, see pages 184 through 191.

Because of the complicated coordination of your entire body, learning to deliver a non-telegraphic punch requires time and sweat. You need to enlist the help of a skilled coach. Words in a book are not going to get it done for you. I can tell you that you need to consciously focus on exploding forward with zero rearward movement. That includes your entire body.

Winding-up Blocks

Yeah, I see it all the time. Martial artists using a wind-up for blocks. I even see instructors teaching a wind-up for blocks. If there was ever a ridiculously counterproductive use of training, this is it. For crying out loud, stop it!

1, Identify Your Telegraphs

This isn't as easy as you might think. While some of our telegraphs are painfully obvious, others are so subtle that we are completely unaware of them. In either case, the most effective way to identify them is to enlist the help of a skilled observer. Your observer will observe from two vantage points, sparring with you and while you spar with someone else. Your observer must know what to look for. Again, this is not as easy as it sounds because there are so many possible ways to telegraph. Becoming familiar with the basic telegraphs in the following section is a good start that you can build upon with experience.

Your observer should first point out the obvious big telegraphs. Later, the observer will focus on your head, then on your shoulders, then your hips, your knees, and your feet. The observer must look for movements as well as telegraphic positions.

This is not a one-time exercise. This will be a process. As we advance in skill, or add new skills, or as our bodies age, we can easily develop new telegraphs. That is why this process should be a part of your training for a lifetime.

A Few Telegraphs To Look For

This is by no means an exhaustive list. This list is intended to get you started on your way to understanding what to look for.

- **Wind-Ups** - Any movement that travels reverse of the intended direction before moving in the intended direction.
- **Eyes** - A very slight glance at your target before striking can be all it takes to alert your opponent of your intentions. Other telegraphs include opening your eyes wider, squinting, or averting your eyes. There are many ways that your eyes can give you away.
- **Facial Expressions** - There are countless facial expressions that can foretell your next move. The old term "poker face" will serve you well when sparring. Grimacing, pursing your lips, furrowing your brow, etc. can all be telegraphs.
- **Favors** - Favoring one body side or a technique can easily telegraph your intention. We all have habits and preferences that give us away. My lead foot kicks typically come from my left. My power kicks come from my right in an orthodox stance, and my spinning kicks come from my left in a southpaw stance. If my opponent picks up on any of these, I will lose some degree of speed.
- **Foot Position** - Problems here are somewhat similar to the wind-up. Many martial artists, especially beginners, will move their

Telegraphing

foot into an unnatural position in preparation for kicking. This is especially prevalent when executing a spinning kick. The kicker will move the trailing foot twelve inches or more into the spin direction expecting it to be easier to execute the kick. This is not only a huge telegraph; it also destroys any chance of proper targeting. Both of these result in tremendous speed loss. Other foot position telegraphs include pulling the foot back before the kick, switching stances, picking the foot up, or any other foot movement that communicates your intentions, especially if repetitive.

- **Hand Position** - Unlike the wind-up, these telegraphs are caused by the position of the hands, or any hand movement, rather than just a wind-up for a strike. Right-hand dominant fighters will often drop their left before throwing the right. Often the hands are thrown out to the sides, an instant before a kick or the hands may both drop just before shooting for a take-down. There are countless hand position telegraphs.
- **Twitches** - While some twitches are obvious, many are nearly imperceptible. The twitch may be on the face, shoulder, fingers, hips, or even the upper legs. These are not only some of the most difficult to detect; they are also some of the most difficult to eliminate.
- **Repetitive Movements** - Any movement that is repeated often enough to make you predictable.
- **Shoulder Movement** - Of course, the shoulder leads in a power strike as do the hips (which lead the shoulder). This does telegraph your strike, but it is not because of poor form that can be corrected. It is part of a proper technique. Shoulder telegraphs occur when the shoulders lead or move when unnecessary for the strike, such as with a jab.
- **Stutter Step** - A martial artist who has poor control of their balance or momentum will often stutter step before executing strikes, kicks, or even defenses.

2. Break The Habits

Most telegraphs are habits, bad habits. They often result from inadequate or poor training. Habits are notoriously difficult to break. I suggest that you work on one telegraph at a time. Once identified, get started on eliminating it. If you have a few similar telegraphs, you can work on them as a group.

Awareness is the first key. Once you've identified a telegraph, remain keenly aware of it. Your speed will suffer during this time because of the conscious thought required, which can cause hesitation. Just like when trying to stop saying "umm" when speaking, you need to catch yourself, and then stop the action. If possible, immediately repeat the scenario in which the telegraph occurred but without the telegraph. Then, repeat it again and again. The goal, as with any training, is to develop a new habit, a desired one.

Setbacks and frustration are a part of attempting to break any habit. Persist. The speed payoff is well worth the effort. Play until you win.

Those Subtle, Nearly Imperceptible Telegraphs

Subtle telegraphs are going to be the most difficult for your observer to identify. That's because they are often perceived subconsciously. That means your observer may be unaware that he or she has detected a telegraph. That doesn't make them any less powerful. In fact, those are often the most powerful telegraphs. Just ask any body language expert, or read a good book on the subject. Intense scrutiny of your observer's actions is required. If your observer repeatedly responds very quickly to a specific attack, without noting a telegraph, it is probable that it is due to subconscious detection of a subtle telegraph. This is why your observer must spar with you.

Subtle telegraphs are often very difficult to eliminate. Because they are subconscious actions, that are often very deeply rooted habits.

3. Use Telegraphs To Your Advantage

Telegraphs can buy you time, and therefore, speed. Whether you're using fake telegraphs to control your opponent or reading your opponent's telegraphs to get early notice of what's coming, telegraphs can be speed gifts.

Acting Class

Make telegraphs pay off. Like a head-fake in football, telegraph-like movements can be used to draw an opening or set up an attack. I call them "telegraph-like" because when used to control your opponent the movements are not telegraphs at all. They are intentional movements that, when done properly, look like telegraphs. They're intended to distract and mislead your opponent. By darting your eyes to the right along with a slight shoulder twitch to the right, you can draw an opening for the left that you intended to throw the entire time. The time that your opponent spends influenced by your faux telegraph is time that adds to your speed. Any telegraph can be used to your advantage to draw your opponent into exposing an opening or committing to a movement that causes a vulnerability.

Use Your Opponent's Telegraphs

Always be on the lookout for any telegraph your opponent commits. Look back at the list of telegraphs above. Those are some of what you are watching for in your opponent. These are speed gifts that should be accepted and exploited vigorously. The more you work on your own telegraphs the better you will recognize telegraphs in your opponents. Train for this to become a subconscious part of your sparring and self-defense. If conscious thought is required, the telegraph will come and go before you will have a chance to take advantage of it. Once mastered, you will attack with speed that will frustrate and confound your opponents. This all comes with training and experience, and then more training and experience. There are no shortcuts.

Control What Your Opponent Hears

When we think about telegraphs, we're usually focused on what we see. What is heard can be just as powerful.

- **Your Breathing** – Never let your opponent hear you breathe. NEVER! Conceal your breathing as much as possible. By hearing your breathing, your opponent can time strikes to maximize damage. Your opponent may understand that most people will not strike on an inhale, which helps them time their attack. Heavy breathing, mouth breathing, or labored breathing tells your opponent that you are gassing out and invites a full assault. You **CAN** train yourself to conceal your breathing even when you are exhausted.
- **Sounds Of Distress Or Pain** – Nothing invites a disabling attack like advertising that you are in distress. Suck it up and stay quiet. You can reel in pain after you win.
- **Sounds That Are Telegraphic** – Any sound that you habitually make that foretells your intentions must be silenced. Grunts, gasps, stomps, whatever, eliminate them.
- **Coaching From Your Corner** – You do know that your opponent can hear everything that you hear, right? If you're going to be coached from your corner, do so in code. Many other sports, like football and baseball, do it, so why shouldn't you? Disinformation is always welcome though.

Great Training For Reading Opponents

Spend a lot of time trying to identify your classmates' telegraphs. This is excellent training for reading opponents. Watch closely when others are sparring. You'll find that even very accomplished martial artists have habits that will telegraph their actions. Some are common among many people, and some are very individual. The more you do this, the quicker and more accurately you will see what others miss. The ability to read your opponent is beyond valuable when pursuing speed.

13

Speed and Power
The speed connection.

WHEN I STARTED STUDYING MARTIAL ARTS, I stood six feet tall and tipped the scales at 132 pounds. When I received my first black belt, I had worked all the way up to 144 pounds. I always knew that power was not going to come easy. Because of that, I focused only on speed and gave power little thought. I used to often say, "I can't hit hard, but I can hit often." That worked well for sparring and point competition, but then I realized that for self-defense, I had to learn to generate power.

I began to look at the physics and body mechanics involved in generating power. I studied boxers in particular. Studying the physics of boxers' punching, I could see that they generated their power by leveraging their contact with the floor along with speed, timing, and full body involvement. While I knew that, due to a lack of mass, I could never have the bone-crushing power of a heavyweight, I soon realized that, by applying my speed to better utilization of body mechanics, I could easily increase my power. That new-found power combined with smart target selection would be much more effective for self-defense, even at my light weight. I now weigh-in at 165 pounds, but I still have to work hard for power.

It's Not Just About Speed, It's Not Just About Power

I would prefer to rely on speed alone because speed comes easier for me due to my slim build. That would be as foolish as a large muscular fighter relying on power alone. Never take the path of least resistance. Train for speed and for power. A heavyweight with speed can be a devastating opponent, but so can a lightweight fighter with power. Regardless of your size, or what comes naturally to you, put in the work to develop both speed and power.

!!! WARNING !!!
The following few sections are the result of a pet peeve of mine. Misuse of "F=ma" to describe how speed creates power bugs me. You are welcome to skip this physics session even though there are a few pieces of useful information hidden within.
Just skip to the bottom of page 183.

F=ma Right? Not So Fast

Martial artists often refer to the formula for Isaac Newton's second law of motion F=ma (force equals mass times acceleration) when speaking of how increased speed also increases power. I've even been guilty of saying it myself. Another phrase, I've heard as long as I can remember is, "speed makes power." Well, it's not that simple. Newton's formula defines forces on an object by multiplying its own mass times its own acceleration. It does not calculate the force exerted on another object with which it collides. Not to mention that speed isn't even in the F=ma formula. Acceleration is, but acceleration is not speed. There is a difference. While we're at it, in the world of physics, power (the kind of power that we want) isn't the same thing as the force in F=ma.

Acceleration is defined as $\Delta v/\Delta t$ (change in velocity divided by change in time). The emphasis here is not on velocity or time, but the rate of change of velocity and time.

Velocity equals change in position divided by time. Velocity is a vector quantity that is direction aware. In other words, velocity has magnitude and a specified direction. I could say that the velocity of a car is 60 mph north. If an object moves constantly but ends up back where it started at the end of the measured time, its velocity is zero because it did not change position for that time period, and therefore, has no direction.

Speed is a scalar quantity which has magnitude only. Speed is defined as distance divided by time. I could say that the speed of a car is 60 mph. An object can go in a circle and end up exactly where it started, and it will still have speed because, unlike velocity, position is irrelevant. The distance traveled and the time required to traverse that distance are the only factors involved.

The force in F=ma is not a resultant force exerted on another object by the mass that is being accelerated. Rather, it is the sum of all forces on the object itself. That doesn't apply to us.

Boxers seem to prefer another formula, P=Fv (power equals force times velocity). Now, we have power and force on opposite sides of the equation. Then, we have velocity which is still not speed. The major problem with this formula is that it calculates average power when a constant force moves an object at a constant velocity (which means in a single direction). Strikes in martial arts are anything but constant by any measure.

Power is the rate at which energy is expended. Power is a scalar quantity meaning that it is not defined by direction. Power can also be defined as the rate of doing work. Still not what we're looking for.

Force is a vector quantity. That means it has direction. This makes sense when we consider another Newton law (his third) that for every action there must be an equal and opposite reaction. That means the forces in play are in opposite directions.

Back To F=ma But, Only To Get To Ft=m Δv

Ft=m Δv should interest you more than F=ma or P=FV. This formula has more to do with collisions and changes in momentum. Those are much more relevant to what we're doing when we strike and block than force and power. Interestingly, we get to Ft=m Δv by way of F=ma.

Remember that the "a" in F=ma is acceleration which is Δv/t (change in velocity divided by time). If we substitute Δv/t in place of "a" in F=ma, it becomes F=m Δv/t. If we multiply both sides of this equation by time, we get Ft=m Δv. This can be put into words as impact force equals mass times the change in momentum. Did "impact force" get your attention? This formula refers to the physics of the impact force of a collision which is what we are interested in. Let's look at the two sides of Ft=m Δv a little closer.

Ft (force times time) is referred to as impulse which is impact force. Impulse is the time span of a collision, hence force times time.

On the other side of our equation, we have m Δv (mass times the change in velocity). We first must know that momentum equals mv (mass times velocity). That means that m Δv equals the change in momentum, which relates directly to the force of a collision.

We now know that impact force (force times time) is equal to the change in momentum (mass times the change of velocity).

We're Still Not There

None of these formulas are adequate for accurately calculating the forces that we apply in martial arts. Primarily that is because these basic formulas require all of the quantities to be constant and they account for only a single constant direction. Virtually nothing is constant when we apply force in martial arts, but that is the payoff. Those variables are what we can take advantage of to generate power by applying what we call "speed."

And Now I Relent... A Little

Okay. The acceleration in F=ma is not speed. Velocity, as in F=Pv, isn't speed either. Intuitively though, we know that if something is moving faster it hits harder. If you throw a bullet at someone, it will bounce off. If you fire that same bullet from a gun... Well, you get the picture. So, we do know that we need to move faster to create more of what we call power, no matter how we define it.

We also intuitively know that a bigger bullet will do even more damage. That is in part because it will carry more momentum. That is where the part about momentum and impact force comes into play. Greater momentum increases impact force because it presents either greater mass or a greater velocity that must be changed (absorbed) by what it impacts.

When we get mass moving by accelerating it to a given velocity, it has momentum which will require force to stop it. The greater the mass and/or the greater the velocity, the greater the momentum, and the greater the force needed to stop it. That force will come from our target as it resists deformation and/or movement during impact.

We'll Call It Speed Anyway

And now that you know what speed isn't, we're going to keep calling it speed anyway. As long as you understand that you must accelerate as quickly and explosively as possible to apply your speed, it doesn't really matter what you call it.

End Of Physics Session

So, What Was The Point Of All Of That Physics Stuff?

You need to look well beyond speed and mass. Speed and mass are very important, but momentum is equally important. Even more important is that you have the ability to control all of the variables involved that those simple formulas don't account for. Your body is a system of levers and force producing muscles that can alter direction, acceleration, velocity, and even mass (the mass involved at the moment). Creating power with the human body is extraordinarily complex. Those complexities are what will be involved in the remainder of this chapter.

By The Way

Calculating the force created by a punch is extremely complicated and defies finite definition due to the multitude of variables involved. Just do a little research on the subject, and you will find that there is nothing even close to a consensus, even among physics experts.

Just A Reminder

This is not a book about power. This is a book about speed, so I'm going to confine most of my points to those that concern speed as it relates to power.

The Power Punch

For the following example, use either a reverse punch, a cross, or a straight punch from your fighting stance.

A punch is used as an example in this section. The purpose is not to teach you how to execute a punch. This is about how to apply speed to increase power. The punch itself is irrelevant. Apply the principles discussed here to other techniques by dissecting them and analyzing them to find every possible way to add speed to them in order to increase their power.

You might find this to be a little anticlimactic. There are no "secrets" to reveal. Applying speed to increase power is mostly about applying speed to components of your techniques that you just may not have before. It is about analyzing your technique and finding every place possible to move faster and then training to make it habit.

1. Power Punch – The Push From The Floor

Power starts at your feet. If you don't believe that, try throwing a power punch while standing on ice. The push from the floor is primarily from your trailing foot. The push is at the toes and ball of the foot. The heel lifts from the floor as your you push forward. The heel also pivots slightly outward to line your foot up with your target. The force created from the push against the floor will be applied through the entire punch and follow through. This is a force variable that simple formulas cannot address as it varies throughout the punch.

Making It Happen

To make this happen faster, your trailing foot must be in position, or at least near position, for the strike at all times. Being flatfooted with your weight on your heels will slow your ability to leverage power from the floor because you must first transition into position. To be fast, you must be light on your feet spending most of your time up on your toes. This puts you in, or at least very near, position for striking with power at all times. Footwork can make or break your speed.

2. Power Punch – Explode Your Leg Extension

The second phase of the power punch is extension of your legs. As your foot braces against the floor, your legs (primarily your trailing leg) extend forcing your upper body forward. Your legs are home to some of the largest muscles in your body. As those muscles work to extend your legs, they can create tremendous force. In addition to the force from your leg muscles, the forward motion of your upper body puts much more of your mass into the punch. This is why mass applied in a strike is difficult to apply in simple formulas. How you execute the punch determines how much of your mass you enlist.

Making It Happen

There are two main factors involved in allowing your legs to create explosive force with speed. First, they must be relaxed. It is impossible to move tense muscles fast. You must train yourself to relax your legs as much as possible while still maintaining stable support. Second, your legs must be slightly bent. Power is created during the extension of your legs (primarily the trailing leg). It is impossible to utilize the power in your legs if your legs are not at least slightly bent. Over bending your knees into a very deep stance can create more power, but at the cost of speed due to the added travel distance required.

Visualization is extremely effective when developing explosive power. When training on the heavy bag, assume your stance, but don't move. Vividly imagine exploding into the punch. You would probably like for me to suggest more detail for the image. Visualization is much more effective if it is based on your perceptions and knowledge base. You need to create the image. I can tell you that it must start entirely calm, and then explode instantly into full force. You may experience results immediately, or it may require a lot of practice. Don't give up too quickly. The power gain that you can achieve is well worth the effort. You may also be a little skeptical of visualization. Whether they talk about it or not, most of the greatest athletes past and present actively use visualization.

3. Power Punch - Hip Rotation

Hip rotation is key to translating power through your torso to your shoulders. Hip rotation happens almost simultaneously with the push from the floor and the leg extension and is aided by the leg extension. Twisting your hips coils your torso like a spring, storing energy that will later be released into your upper body. During this phase of the punch, the hip on your punching hand side moves forward toward your target sharply while the shoulder and arm, on your punching hand side, remain nearly stationary. As your hip moves forward, your core muscles are extended. At the same time, your entire lower body mass is moved forward, and your leg muscles are working to push your body into the direction of your target. The tension created in this motion, in combination with your legs and feet, is where most of your power is created.

Making It Happen

Speed here involves executing the hip rotation as fast as possible. Many power punchers have a habit of moving the hips very slowly. This is in part due to the perception of the power punch being akin to swinging a heavy sledgehammer that slowly swings into position, and then slams its target with lumbering momentum due to its large mass. It can also be due to tension in the legs and core that resists fast movement. It is easy to improve the speed of your hip rotation substantially with a little practice at the heavy bag or when shadow punching. Just throw your punches with good form while concentrating on executing the hip rotation as quickly as possible. You should be as relaxed as possible. This includes your legs, core, arms, and hands. Even tension in your jaw, as I mentioned earlier, can cause tension elsewhere in your body that will slow your movement. Concentrate on relaxing all those areas. The only tension we want is the elongation of the core muscles that will be created by the hip rotation, and the contraction of the muscles developing the push from the floor.

Begin to snap the hip forward. Actively, consciously concentrate on the motion of the hip, and the tension created in your core. In the beginning, don't even throw the punch. Just concentrate on the hip motion (rotation). The greater the tension created, in your core, by the hip rotation the more powerful the punch can be. The faster the hip rotation, the faster the punch can be. An added bonus to fast hip rotation is being less telegraphic because hip rotation is often the first clue to your opponent that the strike is coming.

Be careful to not shorten the hip rotation to make it faster. A shorter hip rotation will yield less power.

4. Power Punch – The Shoulder

During the push from the floor, the leg extension and the hip rotation, the shoulders and arms are relaxed and nearly stationary. They're waiting while your entire body is loading up energy to transfer to them. When your hip reaches full rotation, your core muscles will contract pulling the shoulder of your punching arm forward toward your target. Simultaneously, your shoulder muscles will contract and will begin to pull your arm forward. Your arm must remain as relaxed as possible and will be nearly stationary as the shoulder muscles contract.

Making It Happen

Speed here involves keeping the shoulder relaxed and keeping it in position until just the right time to take full advantage of the energy transfer from your core and legs. A relaxed shoulder can move much faster than a tense shoulder.

Timing of the move forward is all important. Moving the shoulder too soon or too late will negate your power by throwing off the timing of the punch. Moving too early can telegraph your intentions. In either case, speed is lost. Timing of the shoulder movement is learned by practice. You must practice until you become comfortable with your body's timing. Put in time at the heavy bag until proper timing is habit. There are no shortcuts.

5. Power Punch – Arm

The punching arm is next to move. It is propelled forward by the shoulder. It is relaxed until just after the shoulder begins to move it forward. At that time, the agonist muscles in the arm contract to extend the arm, which launches the fist into your target.

Making It Happen

To be fast, the arm must remain relaxed with only adequate isometric tension to maintain its position. The arm itself must remain motionless until time for the agonist muscles to fire. This allows utilization of the premovement silent period discussed in Chapter 4. Train to keep the arm free of extension motion until the moment that the agonist muscles fire. Then, fire them at maximum effort. The contraction must be explosive. The antagonistic muscles of the arm must remain fully relaxed for the duration of the punch. Any tension in the antagonistic muscles will slow the arm extension and will reduce impact force.

6. Power Punch – Wrist

The wrist must be positioned properly for the punch that you've chosen to execute. Use proper form for your style. Weakness in the wrist will negate power and can cause injury. The muscles supporting the wrist must be tensed at impact to transfer power as well as to protect the wrist from injury.

Making It Happen

Keeping the muscles that stabilize the wrist relaxed until impact is the major speed factor.

7. Power Punch – Hand

The hand remains as relaxed as possible during its path toward the target. As with all other body movement, any tension present will detract from your speed. At the moment of contact with your target, the hand must be fully contracted into a fist as tightly as possible.

The contraction of the fist must be timed perfectly for full power transfer into your target. If the hand is too relaxed at contact, it will deform, which will absorb some of the energy. In physics terms, this is called deformability. The more rigid the fist is at contact, the more energy is transferred into the target. Additionally, a fist that is too relaxed at contact will be more easily injured.

Making It Happen

The extension of your arm will provide most of the speed for delivery of your fist to its target. However, the forward motion of your shoulder, torso, and legs will contribute to the speed of your fist as well. This is like throwing a rock forward from a car that is moving forward. The car's speed adds to the speed of the rock because the rock was already moving at the speed of the car. For this reason, you must concentrate on speed as well as power in your legs, torso, and shoulders as well as your arm.

8. Power Punch – Body Drive Forward

This is one of those things that presents variables that those simple formulas discussed at the beginning of this chapter just can't account for. Upon contact, you can drive through your target using all of your musculature from the floor to your hand as you continue to thrust your entire mass forward into the point of impact. You can drive as deeply as is advantageous. Key here is to not allow your trailing foot to lose contact with the floor, as it is critical to continue the push with the foot to maximize your thrust forward into your target. Notice that I did not say, "Push into your target." I said "thrust" into it. Once you begin to just push, you are no longer impacting, and it is time to rechamber, unless you want to attempt to push your opponent in order to effect a takedown or to execute a follow-up technique while your opponent is pushed off balance.

9. Power Punch – When It's Over

This is where you have an opportunity to gain speed that many leave on the table. Just as a batter often lingers at home plate staring at the trajectory of the ball they've just struck, rather than running for first base ala Pete Rose, fighters often linger at the completion of a strike. At the instant that you perceive that you have completed impact, get out or move on instantly. Your next action must happen with the same speed and intensity with which you initiated the strike. Train for this and make it a deep-seated habit.

Speed and Power

Power And Timing

To move fast, you must be as relaxed as possible. To transfer power into your target, you must be as tense as possible. If your hand, wrist, arm, or shoulder are relaxed at impact, it will be akin to hitting your opponent with a wet noodle. Power will not be transferred into your target.

This is very timing critical. That is why this must be trained constantly. This is one of the most difficult things for beginners to learn. Even longtime martial artists sacrifice power due to either being too tense during delivery or poorly timing tension that should occur at the moment of impact. It's similar to whipping a towel. If the snap is not timed perfectly, power will not be transferred into your target. Not to mention that no matter how well you've trained, you won't always get it right because you can't always predict what your opponent will do.

Making It Happen

This is one of those things that you must experience to get it. Spend lots of time at the heavy bag delivering power punches with as much speed and explosiveness as possible. Ensure that your power is not expended too early or too late. You need to end in a stance that will allow you mobility, not overcommitted in any direction. This is a great time to practice rechambering immediately after power is transferred into your target. There's no substitute or trick involved. Just ensure that you are using proper form and practice, practice, practice.

Power Strikes Are Slower

Power strikes are inherently slower than harassment and setup strikes. They are slower because they typically have farther to travel (trailing hand or leg) and require more commitment of body motion. They are also more telegraphic due to the process of storing energy in the core and legs, which requires body movement prior to deployment of the strike itself. Telegraphing gives time, and therefore speed, to your opponent. Before delivering a power strike, ensure that you have a clear opening.

Use A Setup Technique

Because power punches are relatively slow, it is advantageous to use a setup technique or a diversion. This is to reduce the time between when your opponent perceives the strike and when it arrives.

Don't Forget About Blocks

Blocks often require power similar to strikes. They're even more dependent on speed because blocks are in reaction to something that is already happening. That means there is much less time for execution. To save time, and make the blocks stronger at the same time, use blocks with folded limbs. That means a leg check or arm block with the arm folded tightly at the elbow and lying against your body. These blocks are much stronger than extended limb blocks because they make much better use of leverage and larger muscle groups. The downside is that, because your block is held closer to your body, the strike is permitted to get much closer to you. The strike's travel time is longer though which affords you more time to execute the block.

The Speed Habit's Dark Side

Speed can give us the illusion of power. Often when we move fast, we expend a great deal of energy, but we don't connect. We know that many fast techniques, such as snapping techniques, lack power, but it's not just technique selection that causes the problem. It's more of a mindset and perception problem. When we score at will with speed, our perception of what we are doing is that we are effective. If points are all you're interested in, fine, but if self-defense or full contact fighting is your goal, then you've got serious problems. Power requires commitment of motion and commitment in training. Don't neglect training to connect with power. Speed doesn't do a thing for power if all you do is touch.

For self-defense and for full-contact fighting, we train to deliver devastating power with every strike. Those strikes are intended to inflict serious injury. The problem is that, with the exception of full-contact fighters, we train with people that don't want to get hit.

To avoid injuring our training partners, we pull our power. We throw strikes with full speed but pull up the power just before contact with our intended target. If done properly, the striking limb will not be fully extended at contact showing that you could have completed the technique with full power if you had wanted to by completing the extension into the target. This is common in sparring, competition, and self-defense training.

Pulling our power benefits us by allowing us to train at full speed and in dangerous situation simulations. Pulling our power can also lead to big problems. When we train repeatedly, we develop deeply rooted habits. Pulling your power can become a seriously disabling habit. Schools are churning out students that cannot hit with power because it's simply something they never do. Even worse, the students don't even realize it.

My Experience With The Dark Side

For many years, I trained several hours a day for competition sparring in a style where contact was limited. Throwing a strike with full power and speed without damaging contact is as much a skill as anything else that we train for. Speed and precision are required and is developed through serious training. The problem was that I neglected the training needed to actually deliver power into my target. I was so focused on competition that, without even realizing it, I was losing the ability to transfer power into my target.

I began having dreams in which I was attacked by shadowy figures. I would fight back, but no matter how hard I tried I couldn't actually connect a strike. I was fighting furiously, but my punches and kicks all stopped as if my arms and legs were being held back by an unseen force.

Shortly after the dreams started, I was invited to a private match with a fellow competitor at a school he owned. After the match, we talked for a while during which time he told me about dreams he was having that were nearly identical to mine. It was at that moment that I changed my training to ensure that I could actually connect with power when needed.

Training For Power

Train for form first. Don't add power or speed until your form is correct and efficient. Let me emphasize that. You will be wasting your time and accomplishing nothing worth having if you are working on speed and power while using incorrect or inefficient form. You'll just solidify bad habits, setting yourself up for failure, and increasing your risk for injury.

Hit People

There is no substitute for actually making contact. It is impossible to develop the timing and distance control necessary to reliably strike with power without contact sparring. Unfortunately, it's becoming a thing of the past. Most schools allow only light contact sparring. This is because of liability issues, and the fact that if they allowed heavy, or even medium, contact they would be lucky to have four students. Some schools don't even allow sparring at all, which is just tragic.

If you are fortunate enough to get some sparring time in, make the most of it. Spar as many opponents as possible. Everyone's timing and distance control is different. Become as versatile as possible. As a bonus, you get to learn how to take a hit. That is a skill just like any other.

Gear up heavily and spar heavily. It is the only way to ensure that you can connect with speed and power against an actual opponent. A full complement of gear is required including headgear and large, heavily padded gloves.

14

Skills and Training
A box full of speed.

SPEED IS NOT A SUBSTITUTE FOR EFFECTIVE FORM. No matter how fast you become, always use effective technique. Even if it means slowing down to do it. Nothing matters more than getting the job done effectively. Notice that I didn't say "proper" form. The technique might be considered proper for your style, but that doesn't mean it is effective. If you seriously practice poor, ineffective technique, you may become faster, but you will not be fast because you will never reach effective completion. You can stay within your limits and be effective, or you can move as fast as possible and hope for the best.

Making It Happen
- Before anything else, you need to know if the technique is effective. Evaluate the technique. Take the time to fully understand it. You may find that it is just a decorative technique that has no real application to your goals. If so, don't bother training it for speed. Abandon it now.
- Ensure that your execution of the technique is effective. Know

exactly how it should be executed (that may or may not be how you've been shown). Know its intended targets, the most efficient route for execution, when it should be utilized, the best hip position, etc. Don't train for speed until you know exactly what you need to do. Understand the details. Then, adapt the technique to you and your body.
- Train for form and do it slowly. Always train for form first and speed second. You know, walk before you run. Practice enough to be able to reliably execute the technique. A thousand or so reps (with effective form) is a good start.
- Then and only then should you begin to practice with speed. Add speed constantly, but always with effective execution foremost on your mind.

You'll Thank Me Later

Here's a challenge for you. Pick a kick that is already on your go-to list. It must be effective, so pick one that you know can score. Add a setup technique if needed. I prefer the simple, uncool kicks like the front kick.

Now, spend the next few weeks training that kick until you start doing it in your sleep. Focus your training for perfection. Keep in mind that you're training for exceptional speed, not just general oh-look-I'm-a-little-faster speed. Work that technique until it snaps out before you even know that you're going to do it. Train until it is a part of you.

Making It Happen
- Give it as many reps as possible every day. A hundred reps is a reasonable start, but more would be better.
- When you're too tired to practice, physically train in your mind. When you practice in your mind, the same neural pathways fire that fire when it's real. There is a lot of science to back up the effectiveness of vividly practicing in your mind. Do it, and then do it a lot more.

Skills and Training

- Don't vary the target. If you're planning on sticking it in your opponent's gut, see it going exactly there every rep. At the heavy bag, put it there every rep.
- Visualize it working every rep. See it and experience it in your mind. Sink that technique as deeply in your mind as possible.
- Practice with your hands in chamber. You should have no need whatsoever for your hands or arms as ballast.

After six weeks or so, put it to work in your sparring. You already know what's going to happen. Now, get started on another technique.

Sparring: Order The Opening That You Want

Most sparring is a continuous exchange of initial attacks. Initial attacks create openings. Bait your opponent into initiating the attack that you want, and you get the opening that you want. Knowing where to counterattack can get you there tremendously faster.

Get Rid Of A Bunch Of Techniques

That old saying, "Jack of all trades, master of none" offers a lot of power to anyone who will take it to heart.

I believe you can be a dominant competitor even if you limit your kicking arsenal to only three kicks. In fact, I believe you can dominate using only your left leg. Let's go a step further and limit you to only lead foot kicks. That's a very slim kick selection.

Now, let's add in that every competitor you meet knows ahead of time exactly which three kicks you are limited to along with knowing which foot is going to deliver them. They even know that they will all come off the lead foot. I still believe that you can not only dominate I believe that you can compete full contact and knock out half of your opponents on your way to a perfect professional record. If you disagree with that, tell Bill "Superfoot" Wallace. That's exactly what he did.

Bill "Superfoot" Wallace is a retired Professional Karate Association (PKA) full-contact fighter. Due to an injury, Wallace suffered early in his martial arts career, he was limited to kicking with only his left foot. He used only three kicks, all with the lead foot. All three kicks were incredibly fast. When you stepped into the ring with Wallace, you not only knew exactly what kicks were coming, you knew which side they were coming from. Unfortunately, there was very little that you could do about it. The poor fellow only racked up 23 wins and ZERO losses in his pro career.

Wallace MASTERED those three kicks. Kicks would often hit his opponents before they even realized that they were coming. He's now 71 years old (at the time of this writing), and what do you know? He can still deliver those kicks better, and faster, than most accomplished 20-year-old martial artists and with incredible flexibility for any age.

Do you get the point? Mastering a few solidly effective techniques is tremendously more useful than being halfway proficient with a hundred. This is a direct path to being devastatingly fast. Get rid of the fluff. Experts specialize. Become an expert.

Use A Single Kicking Chamber

Use a single chamber for as many kicks as possible. I mean chamber them identically. It is extremely effective and it's easy. A single chamber has many advantages. It simplifies and enhances your training simultaneously. That single chamber gets trained no matter what kick you're practicing. Therefore, it gets a lot of reps and becomes darned fast.

A single chamber is very deceptive. Your opponent finds out very late exactly what kick is coming because all the way through the chamber, they all look identical. I read recently that Bill Wallace credited a lot of his success to the use of a single chamber (his was very different than mine), so we're in very good company.

Making It Happen

This is how I chamber. It makes sense for my body and my fighting style. Use this as an example. It will be up to you to adjust and adapt this concept to your body and your fighting style.

For any non-spinning kick, I chamber by bringing the knee straight up in front of me with my lower leg perpendicular to the floor in what looks like a knee lift movement. In the case of a trailing leg kick, my kicking foot passes very close to my support leg. It's as simple as that.

Every kick that I deliver leads with the knee and completes in a single motion. I use no exaggerated hip or support foot rotation. Both of those cause overcommitment of motion that will reduce recovery speed and mobility. Although a deep chamber typically translates to a fast and powerful kick, you still should chamber the knee only as high as necessary. Chambering too high often turns the kick into a two-step movement with a slight pause at the peak of the chamber. This is slow and unnecessary. Chambering too high also slows the kick as it adds wasted motion.

I use the same chamber for spinning kicks, although it is a little more complicated. The main difference is the trajectory of my knee. In non-spinning kicks, the primary movement of my knee is upward. Some forward trajectory is involved depending on where the kick is going. For spinning kicks, the knee is lifted during the rotation (as late as possible). For a spinning hook to the head, the chamber is high with the knee traveling in an arc parallel to the floor. For a back kick, the knee travels a straighter line to its target. In either case, the chamber is as late as possible and as shallow as possible. As shallow as possible doesn't mean that you should never use a deep chamber. It means that you don't chamber deep when a shallow chamber is sufficient.

Wallace used a very different kicking chamber than most fighters because he didn't use a typical boxer-style fighting stance. His stance was closer to a shallow horse-riding stance.

Kick In One Motion

When teaching kicks, we instructors emphasize the chamber, and then the execution of the kick. Beginners often get the idea that the kick should be executed in two distinct steps. Yeah, there are two parts, but there is only one kicking motion.

Making It Happen

I talk a lot about chambering, but that doesn't mean you should ever linger there. The chamber and completion of the kick is always one smooth, uninterrupted motion. Most kicks lead with the knee. Use that. The knee comes up fast and hard toward its target as a vehicle for the lower leg, which whips out loose and fast with no tension until the moment of impact when the entire kick culminates with power transferred from your entire body.

To Kick Fast, Chamber Fast

Unlike hand techniques, kicks must move to chamber before executing. That makes the kicking chamber motion extremely important to your speed. You must chamber as fast as possible. The speed of the chamber dictates the speed of the entire kick and determines when your opponent knows that a kick is on its way.

Making It Happen

Train your chamber during every training session. Because your chamber heavily involves your core, and doesn't unduly tax your knees or hips, it can be trained more than kicks. Train it during your warm-up, during your cooldown, for cardio, or any other time you train. The most important thing is to always chamber explosively and with proper form. Mix it up too. Chamber high, low, and for spinning kicks.

Skills and Training

Knees, Elbows, And Uppercuts For Inside

Knees, elbows, and uppercuts lack reach, but when you are very close to your opponent, they can be both fast and devastating. Each of these techniques can be thrown effectively with very short travel, so they are powerful close range weapons. To be fast when working inside, stick to short, but powerful, techniques.

If It's Fancy, It's Probably Slow

I used to love fancy, complicated kicks. They pack great wow factor at demonstrations, they're fun, they make for a great workout, they're great for improving balance and body control, and they have no place whatsoever in sparring or self-defense. This goes for fancy or complicated hand techniques, footwork, stances, or anything else that is inefficient and slow. To be fast, leave these for show time.

Your Defense Needs To Be Faster Than Your Offense

If you are defending, your opponent moved first, and a weapon is already on its way. That head start means you've got to be very fast to evade or stop what's coming. To be effective, you must train your defense as intensely as you train your offense, with emphasis on making it happen fast. Here are some keys to fast defense:

- **Train for fast perception.** The earlier you perceive what's coming, the more time you will have to do something about it. See Chapter 3.
- **Use minimal movement.** Your blocking and evasion movements must be very efficient. Move only as much as necessary. See Chapter 7.
- **Eliminate tension.** Relaxing when being attacked can be difficult. Come to terms with it. See "Pain" (page 220) and "Enjoy Getting Hit" (page 158).
- **Use effective blocks.** Touching isn't blocking.
- **Slip what you can.** Slips require much less movement.
- **If it's going to miss, don't block it.** You're wasting motion.

Keep Your Dang Hands Up!

To be fast your hands need to be where they are useful. Not some of the time, ALL OF THE TIME. If they have to travel to get back to a useful position before you can use them, you've given away speed. That means when you are kicking too. Actually, especially when you are kicking. You might think that an outstretched arm over your side kick looks cool, but it doesn't. It tells me that you want to eat a counter kick in the ribs and that you have no plans to use that hand for anything other than ballast. This also doesn't mean just when you're sparring. I mean all the darn time. Develop this habit to the point that you have to be told to put them down. The only time, during sparring, that your hands should leave useful position is when they are doing something useful.

Instructors and upper belt students should constantly remind lower belts to keep their hands up so that they develop the habit early. When I'm partnered with a lower belt for kicking drills, I tell them to call me out if I drop my hands. Who cares that I'm a black belt?

When You're Fast, You May Need To Drop Your Hands

When I was competing, I spent a lot of time with my hands straight down by my sides. Sometimes, I even put them behind my back. That is because I'm a counter fighter. I prefer that my opponent moves first. Once your opponent realizes how fast you are, they are typically reluctant to attack. You will need to draw your opponent in. This tactic works best if you can appear tired or like you just don't know what you're doing. Appear a little off balance or intimidated. It's a trap, so use attractive bait. This doesn't violate my rule of keeping your hands up because you are using your hands for good purpose.

Never Kick Like The Figure On Top Of Your Trophy

Really. The lady's and the men's trophies are both embarrassing. Who the heck designed those things? I just had to get that one off my chest.

Understand

Change your approach to day-to-day training. Never just practice. Dissect your technique. Understand every single part of the technique. If you want to be exceptional, develop exceptional understanding of what you are doing.

Start with the basics. That is where you build the foundation that will support speed. Don't even think about working on fancy or advanced techniques until you have truly mastered your stances, footwork, punches, basic kicks, and blocks, or whatever makes up the basics of your chosen art. Once you've mastered them, practice them even more.

Does this sound boring? Does being exceptional sound boring? Does commanding outstanding speed sound boring? Do a little research on the greatest athletes in all sports. A common thread you will find among the greatest of the great is mastery of the basics. They did the boring work, and then they did it more than almost anyone. That is where their seemingly superhuman skills came from.

When Speed Makes You Slow

In my prime, I had a very fast double side kick. Maybe too fast. The plan was for me to flick the first one (a fake) down low, and then, while their attention was still down low, I would land the second one on their head.

In martial art schools, you will encounter a wide variety of opponents. I began to realize that my opponents fell into one of three categories.
1. Those who were oblivious to fakes.
2. Those who never see fakes because they happen too fast.
3. Those who will fall for fakes.

So, part of the time my fake was a wasted effort because my opponent was too unskilled to even know to be concerned about it. Other times I executed the fake so quick that it was never seen. I realized that the end result for both of these was that I ended up (in my opponent's view) just executing a slow side kick. At least it wasn't as fast as it could have been if I hadn't wasted my time with the unseen fake. Sometimes you're faster if you slow down a little. Execute that fake slow enough for it to be seen and effective. Or, you could just forego the fake.

Another Time That Speed Makes You Slow

My favorite point sparring kick is my spinning hook. I'm a headhunter with it, and I throw it very fast. This is great if heavy contact is okay or if the sparring breaks on points. If neither of these is the case, I'm required to control the kick. I also must control the kick if I'm sparring a lower belt student lest I take someone's head off.

So, I throw the kick to the head and take great care to stop short in order to protect my sparring partner. Again, this is fine if we're breaking on points. However, if the sparring is continuous, my opponent will invariably take advantage of me while my foot lingers by their head because I was protecting them. The result is that the fast kick ends up being slow, and I pay the price for it by being countered. You might be thinking that your opponent should acknowledge the point and your protective pause. From experience, I'll tell you to not count on it.

Blocking

Blocking is the act of placing a less vital body part in the path of an attack to protect a more vital or more vulnerable body part. Blocks are very dependent on perception, response, fast movement, and accuracy. Because blocks are defensive techniques, by definition, you will be the second one to move. This puts you behind in every category.

Blocks are also dependent on power. In typical martial art schools, sparring blocks are often little more than touches. A touch is sufficient when the sparring is very controlled. Touching is a waste of movement and time unless you think it is necessary to avoid having a judge award a point against you. Touching is obviously not enough for full-contact sparring or self-defense. To deliver an effective block against an unrestrained attack, power sufficient to stop or deflect the attack is necessary. Power requires commitment of motion. Ensure that you maintain your body position and balance.

> Block as fast as you strike!
> Block as fast as you strike!
> BLOCK AS FAST AS YOU STRIKE!!!
> *Am I making my point?*

Using Your Elbows and Forearms For Faster Blocks

Most martial artists block their body with their hands. This takes their hands out of chamber, which typically leaves their head vulnerable to strikes. Blocking kicks to the midsection and lower body this way is very slow because of the distance that the hand must travel.

Elbows and forearms are much faster. Assume that you are in a boxing type chamber. Blocking kicks or strikes to your midsection requires no more than a shift of the forearm or elbow and maybe a little torso pivot. Your hands remain where they are and ready to protect your head or to execute an attack. This type of blocking is extremely fast, effective, and requires very little movement, which reduces arm fatigue.

Because elbow and forearm blocks allow strikes to get very close your body, they may not be advisable for tournament sparring. It's difficult for judges to determine if a strike scored, or if it was blocked when it gets that close. This can cause you to give up points. For tournament sparring, it may be better to give the judges a big block to see.

The Backfist Is Not As Fast As A Jab

I'm in danger of martial art blasphemy here. Many martial artists believe the backfist to be the fastest strike available. The jab is actually much faster. The jab takes a very direct, straight-line route to its target. It's the fastest punch available to you.

As it's most often executed, the backfist takes an angular and arcing approach to its target, which is a longer path than the jab takes. The arcing path makes sense because the target for the backfist is most often the side of the head. To put a snap on the end of the backfist, the arm must reverse direction before impact. That creates a small delay before impact as the forearm reverses direction. Of course, you can deliver the backfist without the snap at the end for a little more speed. It is also possible to throw the backfist in a straight path. It's just rarely executed that way. In fact, most often (almost always) the backfist is thrown after being pulled across the body in a wind-up motion before it begins its forward travel. That wind-up adds substantial time and increases the distance and arc on its way to its target. It also makes the strike very telegraphic.

The jab can also be executed with a flick of the wrist for added power, but with no loss of speed. It's just rarely seen. It's still a straight-line technique, and the wrist motion is less pronounced and directed into the target along with the momentum of the arm instead of pulling the arm rearward. This is faster than the backfist wrist motion. Muhammad Ali routinely threw this jab with incredible power.

In support of the backfist is the fact that, for many martial artists, it is a very natural strike to deliver. That facilitates speed. Then, there's the fact that many martial art styles leave the side of the head vulnerable to the backfist. That means it still may be the fastest choice for you. Or at least, fast enough. It's your choice. Or, you could become proficient with both the backfist and the jab.

It seems nearly everyone likes to throw the backfist from an arm that is hanging in front of them with the fist just above the knee. This greatly increases the travel distance and is just a lousy place to position your arm for defense. To be fast, keep your hands up.

Skills and Training

The Jab

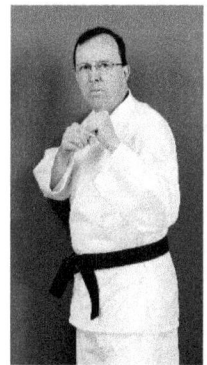 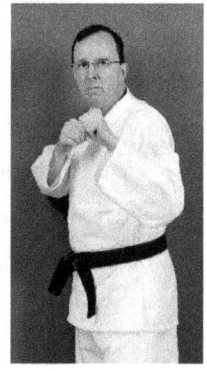 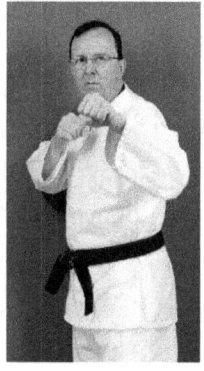 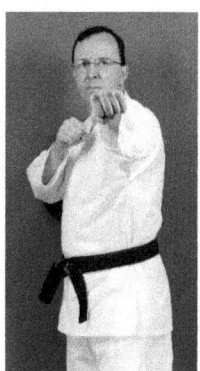

The jab travels a very straight, efficient path to its target.

The Backfist

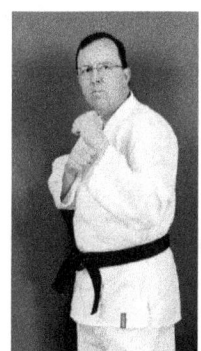 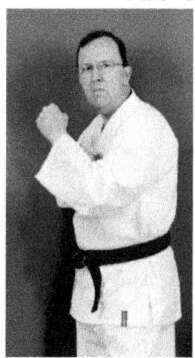 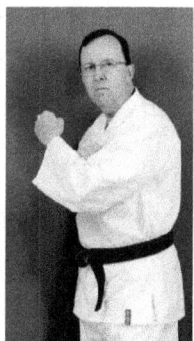 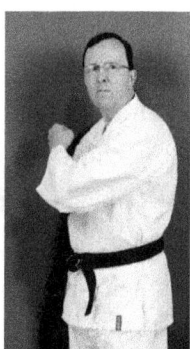

Most often the backfist is pulled across the chest before execution.

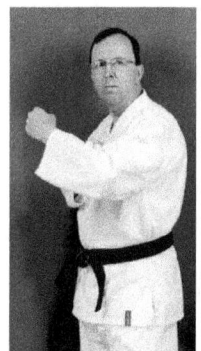 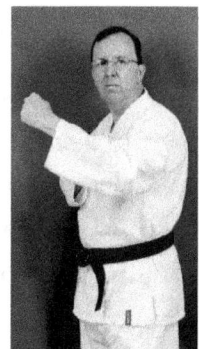 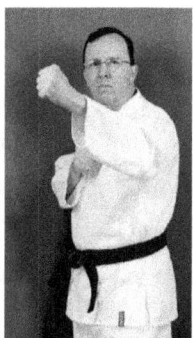 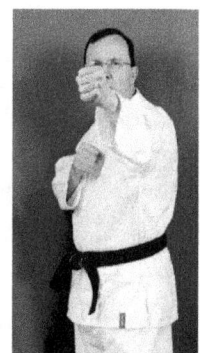

The backfist travels an arcing, angular approach to its target.

Never Lead With A Spinning Kick

Really. Why do I even need to say this? Because I see it happen constantly. That's why. There are many competition styles in which spinning kicks can be effective. Leading with a spinning kick, though, never provides a speed advantage. You may get away with leading with a spinning kick from time to time, but it isn't because of a speed gain. Spinning kicks need to be executed as part of a combination, as a follow-up technique, or as a counter to be effective.

Strategy

So, what does strategy have to do with speed for the martial artist? Strategy is nothing more than a plan to achieve something. Strategy requires making decisions concerning your actions prior to the event. If you make your decisions during the event, time for conscious thought is required. Time is the measure of speed. Responding based on prior training and decisions requires little or no conscious thought or time. The more efficient and effective your strategy is, the quicker your goal is achieved. Take your time formulating your strategy in as much detail as possible. Make that strategy a part of you by rehearsing mentally often. That is the path to speed of execution. Of course, strategies often meet a quick death in the presence of reality, so stay adaptable.

Long Range Strategies

Strategies for the martial artist can take many forms. For sport martial artists, where there are strict rules, developing a strategy may require intensive planning where the strategy is part of a precisely planned and executed training regimen that is strongly influenced by the rules of the contest. Strategy development may include detailed study of the opponent, including review of video of past matches. The knowledge gained would be integral to strategy and training for the contest. In this case, the strategy would include ways to exploit the opponent's weaknesses and avoid the opponent's strengths. The rules of the contest can greatly affect strategy development. Training to the point that functioning within the confines of the rules becomes subconscious will eliminate the need for conscious thought. This allows the martial artist to compete at peak speed with no need for conscious thought.

Don't Let Your Opponent Start Over

Disengaging after every encounter allows your opponent to reset. Any speed advantage that you may have had as a result of your opponent's lack of balance, commitment of motion, or failure to rechamber is lost. Most sparring happens like it's happening on a balance beam. One competitor kicks or punches a few times while the other retreats in a straight line. Then, they swap roles, and the other competitor walks the beam backward. Repeat, repeat... Time your counterattack and then pressure. Use advancing angular movement to evade attacks while placing you in position to score. Mix up your timing to confuse your opponent. Anything that puts you closer to your target or creates an opening is speed gained. Only disengage when absolutely necessary in order to put you back where you have an advantage.

Being Unpredictable

If your opponent can time you, you are owned. Even if you are moving fast, your speed is reduced. Remember that our speed is measured by the time from when our opponent knows that something's coming and when it gets there. If your opponent predicts accurately, you have lost speed by the fact that your movement was known earlier.

Distraction For Sparring

Distracting your opponent is an excellent way to increase their perception time. You want to cause your opponent to consciously think, to be baited into wasted movement, to move to a position that puts them at a disadvantage, to divert their attention, etc.

As always, the skill and experience level of your opponent will dictate how susceptible he or she is to distraction, but everyone is to some degree. Here are just a few examples of effective distractions:

- Fakes.
- Setups.
- Sounds – Verbal, slapping your leg, stomping the floor.
- Harassment – Jabs, backfists, hitting their gloves.
- Unorthodox or unexpected movement.
- Changing your timing or speed.
- Changing stance or lead.
- Constant movement.
- Appearing incapable of defending.
- Dropping defenses (on purpose to draw an opening).
- Being predictable on purpose.
- Averting your eyes.
- Extending a hand as bait.
- Appearing intimidated.
- Anything that frustrates.

Setups For Spinning Techniques

Spinning techniques, such as spinning kicks and spinning backfists can be very effective for sparring and competition. To make them very fast, use the natural spinning motion of your upper body during the setup technique.

When executing punches, the upper body naturally pivots on its center axis (the spine). This is one reason that straight-line techniques require so much practice. Straight-line movement is much less natural.

Assume that you are standing in a right-foot lead fighting stance, and you intend to attack with a left-hand spinning backfist. A logical setup technique would be any right-hand technique that has a right-to-left trajectory (from your point of view). As the setup arrives at its target, your body is already partially into the pivot needed for the spinning backfist. This approach is very efficient and much faster than using a straight-line setup. A straight-line setup would cause a slight delay between arrival of the setup at its target and initiation of the spin required for the spinning backfist. This setup will work just as well for any left-foot spinning kick.

You can easily substitute a right-foot roundhouse for the setup and achieve the same effect as described above for the left-hand spinning backfist or left-foot spinning kick. It's a little slower than setting up with a hand technique because of the travel time required for your foot to make its way back to the floor after the roundhouse kick.

I typically throw my setup several times in succession with a little less speed than I would use if actually trying to connect. I even tend to let it linger a moment when it reaches full extension. I try to get its presence (typically at head level) firmly fixed in my opponent's mind. When the time is right, I throw the setup with just a little more speed. Just as my setup nears its full extension, I execute a spinning back kick with full speed and commitment into my opponent's midsection.

Of course, there are countless variations that can be used effectively. The best ones for you are the ones that are within the confines of your style or rules, that work well with your body type, and that take advantage of your skillset.

Combinations

Nothing showcases speed like a sudden combination of two, three, or more effective strikes. Throughout this book, I've suggested the use of setup techniques many times. Those are combined techniques, but they're not combinations. The difference is that the first technique is not intended to score. Combinations are multiple techniques thrown in succession that all have the potential to score.

Combinations are fertile ground for a fast fighter. Not only can a fast fighter execute multiple techniques with demoralizing speed, they can also better deal with the downsides of combinations. Combinations are very demanding of stamina due to the greater physical exertion they require. Hand technique combinations can cause you to lose your guard because both hands are busy at nearly the same time. Kicking combinations can severely commit your body motion and can leave you vulnerable to counterattack or being taken down. Below are some things to remember when throwing combinations.

- **Targeting** – Ensure that you have a target for every technique in a combination.
- **Rechambering** – Combinations require fast and efficient rechambering. Rechamber as fast as you strike.
- **Power** – Power is easily lost in combinations. Don't move so fast that you fail to expend power into your target.
- **When** – It's best to execute a combination when your opponent is very vulnerable to ensure that you have the necessary time for effective completion.
- **How many?** – Two strike combinations can, and should, be thrown often. Save the three and four strike combinations for exceptionally opportune times when you have plenty of gas in your tank and your opponent is very vulnerable.

15

Speed for Self-Defense

The most important reason to be fast.

SPEED NEVER MATTERS MORE THAN IT DOES FOR self-defense. Because you're defending, you're the second to move (well, not always). You're even going to be the second one to know that something is going to happen. That means you are starting with a severe speed deficit. Then, there's the fact that your life may be on the line, which means your mind is going to be consumed with conscious thought. You'll also be fighting the debilitating effects of excess adrenaline. You've got to move fast, and you've got to move effectively.

A Few Cautionary Words of Wisdom

There are countless opinions about what constitutes effective self-defense. They vary by martial art style and by instructor. I'm not sure I've ever seen a martial art school that didn't teach "the ultimate in self-defense." Unfortunately, much of the self-defense that is taught in martial art schools is absolutely useless. Worse, a lot of it is dangerous. Not to your attacker, to you. When choreography and fancy moves meet a drug-inspired, desperate attacker who places no value on your life, choreography and fancy moves won't last two seconds. Grapplers tend to fare better, but their advantage goes out the window if there are multiple attackers or if they've failed to add finishing moves to their skillset. A false sense of security is extremely dangerous. So, I implore you to do everything possible to ensure that you are training practically and effectively. That's a tall order considering all the misinformation, unqualified instructors, and myths that abound in the world of self-defense instruction.

Use your own mind. If the techniques you are being taught require the cooperation of your attacker, choreography, or memorization of a script, what you are being taught will be useless in the street.

From The Speed Perspective

I'm going to do my best to confine the content here to the implications of speed on self-defense and how to effect speed in self-defense. My intent is to cover information you may not have heard before and that has a profound impact on your speed.

> ### The Definition Of Speed For Martial Artists
> *"The time that elapses from perception to effective completion."*

1. Decisions

Up 'til now, I've told you over and over that conscious thought is slow. Well, now I'm telling you that it's fast. In fact, conscious thought is the fastest weapon you have for self-defense. It can easily be the difference between life and death.

Speed for Self-Defense

Most people have no clue what they will do in a self-defense situation. That's because they've never given it a thought. Brilliant. Wait until your life is on the line, and you've got adrenaline flowing by the gallon to decide what you're going to do. Yeah, that should turn out just great. Even most martial artists haven't thought past how they envision smashing anyone who dares to take them on.

Making your decisions ahead of time can make you so fast that you win without ever even fighting. That's right. You can win without moving a muscle. If you are forced to fight, the decisions you make now will massively increase your speed and chances of winning. The conscious thought you put into these decisions now will reduce your need for conscious thought when you must defend yourself. Not only will you make better choices in the moment, you will also be able to act much faster.

You're likely thinking I've made some bold claims here. Well, I've actually understated it. If you turn off your ego and engage your brain, you can up your self-defense ability beyond measure.

The *FASTEST* Self-Defense Technique In Existence

Don't be there. That's right. If you think that there might be trouble, don't go. Wow, that was a letdown, wasn't it? Not really. You see, often we know when there is going to be trouble. So, decide to not be there. But, martial arts is about fighting. I'm a black belt, and you're telling me to be a wimp? Being smart isn't being a wimp. Martial artists fight only when they are forced to. It's not about how tough you are. It's about staying safe. So, make the smart choice. When you can avoid trouble, do it.

How can you make self-defense any faster than not having to defend yourself in the first place? That is the ultimate in speed for self-defense, and it should be your primary goal no matter how right you are or how well you can fight.

Do You Want To Fight, Or Do You Want To Win?

Stay with me here, this is going to get to speed. This question came to me one day when I desperately wanted to give someone a piece of my mind. The problem was that I needed this person on my side for other purposes. Chewing them out would give me short-term satisfaction and a small win, but it was going to hand me a huge long-term loss. Biting my tongue was one of the toughest things I've ever done, but to win, I had to smile and endure their mindless crap. The only way to tolerate the situation was to constantly remind myself that losing this small battle was going to win the war for me in the end.

I'm sure that you want to win. That's what we train for. The problem is that often what we consider winning just digs us in deeper. If we want to win, we need to define what winning is. For self-defense, I define winning as going about my life the way I want to unharmed and not in jail. That means I will avoid a fight if at all possible. I know, that's not very macho. We, martial artists, train to fight. So, why the heck should I put in all that training time and then not fight? We train to fight so that we win when violence is thrust upon us, and we are left with no other choice.

There are lots of people who had good reason to fight and who won their fight and are still living behind bars. If they're honest about it, many of them will tell you they could have avoided the fight. Many of them knew better than to even be where the trouble started in the first place. And, they probably let their ego prevent them from avoiding trouble once it started. Ask them if you're a wimp for not fighting. You sometimes have only microseconds to decide whether or not to fight. The courts have years to decide if they think that you were justified. And, they don't always get it right.

Decide To Win

That means avoiding the fight if all possible and it means fighting to win if you are forced to fight. See "When It's Time To Fight" below.

Speed for Self-Defense

Let Me Be Clear

I'm not telling you to put yourself in danger by hesitating, and therefore, putting yourself at a disadvantage. I'm telling you to not be boneheaded stupid and dive into a fight that you clearly could have avoided. Ego, meaningless arguments, and the protection of physical belongings do not justify fighting. I'm trying to protect you. Martial artists sometimes get stuck in the fight mindset. I like fighting as much as any of you reading this. I detest bad guys as much as any of you. I just know that fighting must remain a last resort for many reasons. More on this in the section on fighting below.

Need A Little More Incentive To Not Fight?

Dang! I just won't get off of this don't fight stuff will I? Well, it's that important, and I still believe it's the fastest way to victory. Just consider these questions for me, and I'll stop: Do you really want the legal trouble? Do you want to swap bodily fluids with this person? You do know that you may lose, right? Do you want what may come with that? Remember that bad guys tend to come in bunches, and they gang up just for the fun of it. Even if you win, you probably won't come away unharmed. Got your kids or some other vulnerable person with you? What happens to them when you dive into a fight that you could have avoided? Can you afford to be out of work for a few weeks? Have you got the extra bucks around for a lawyer? Yeah, in our society you can be totally in the right and still spend a fortune trying to prove it.

My Self-Defense Continuum

1. If you think that there's going to be trouble, don't go.
2. If you get there and it looks like trouble, leave.
3. If you are there and trouble comes to you, get away if possible.
4. Give them what they want (within reason). But, never drop your guard.
5. Never let anyone transport you. Period.
6. If you have no other choice, fight to win.

Heel-toe, heel-toe...

In self-defense classes, I often start with what I call the heel-toe, heel-toe method. Now keep in mind that your typical self-defense class student is expecting to learn how to break bones and disarm gun-wielding bad guys. To teach them the heel-toe, heel-toe method I extend my left foot and place my heel on the floor. Moving forward, I rock that foot up onto its toes and extend my right foot forward and place its heel on the floor. I then rock the right foot up onto its toes and repeat the left foot movement. Simultaneously, I'm saying "heel-toe, heel-toe, heel-toe..." I'll add that the faster you do it, the better it works. What I've just demonstrated is running. Now, I'm not actually saying that you should always run. My intent is to move their mindset from a fight only mindset to one of avoidance and options. And, fighting only when there is no other choice.

Decide What You Are Willing To Do To Win A Fight

Those who prey on the innocent often have no inhibitions about inflicting great bodily harm or even taking someone's life. Whether you believe it or not, you do have limits. To overcome an assailant, you're going to need to be brutal. Are you sure that you can claw someone's eyes, break their bones, or choke them unconscious? Can you actually take someone's life? Don't just give me a "heck yeah!" and read on. Tougher people than you have struggled with these decisions and the aftermath of carrying them out. Deal with it now as honestly and thoroughly as possible. On one hand, it can save your life by eliminating hesitation, which is death to speed. On the other hand, it may prevent you from doing something rash that you will ultimately regret.

Squeamish?

While we're on the subject of what you are willing to do, let's talk about being squeamish. Fighting can be a messy business. Not everyone has the stomach to do what is necessary to stop an attacker. Effective self-defense techniques break bones, tear flesh, and can involve blood and gore. While none of us want any of this, we need to be prepared for it.

Just the act of viewing a mental image of the possibilities can serve to desensitize you. If images like this are thrust upon you without preparation, the shock can be debilitating. The result can go beyond hesitation and head straight to deer-in-the-headlights paralysis. For self-defense, you must be able to act without hesitation. Do whatever it takes for you to reduce your emotional responses to what you may see or need to do to protect yourself. See "Is There A Nurse In the House?" (page 155).

Pain

Decide now to deal with pain. No matter how effective your fighting skills are, you're probably going to get hurt. You can't be fast if you're preoccupied with pain. Deal with it now. If you are fighting for your life, or the life of others, you don't stop for pain, you don't acknowledge pain, and you don't think about pain. You just fight. Pain isn't going to hurt you. Yeah, I meant to say that. Letting pain prevent you from doing what's necessary to protect you, will get you really hurt.

Making It Happen

As a martial artist, you've probably got this. You've already dealt with a lot of pain in training. If not, find some. That's right. Do something that hurts (within reason) and deal with it. Workout to the point of pain and then push further. Spar with enough contact to hurt a little. Do some breaking. Find a safe way to learn to deal with pain. Mentally come to terms with pain.

Avoid Self-Inflicted Pain

Many instructors teach striking the head with a closed fist and knuckle contact. I think that is a bad idea. If you wrap a one-inch-thick piece of foam around a bowling ball and slug it with all you've got (**don't actually do this**), how much of your hand do you expect to not be broken? That's about the equivalent of slugging a skull. Sure, you can get away with a punch to the head with a well-placed shot to the jaw or nose, but can you really count on that much accuracy? To be fast and effective, your weapons must be intact, and it's best if you're not reeling in pain. For headshots, I prefer the palm-heel, elbow, or forearm. You do lose distance, which loses speed, but you gain the ability to strike again. You can't be fast if you're out of the fight.

Decide What You Will Do

Most people have no clue what they will do if they are forced to defend themselves. This is a major speed disadvantage. It means you're going to be forced to make those decisions when there is no time and you are at the peak of stress. Make your decisions ahead of time. How will you fight? Will you fight at all? What are you willing to do? What weapons (fists are weapons) will you use? How will you use them? Run scenarios through your mind. You will discover more decisions that need to be made. Make all of them that you can.

I'm not suggesting that you script any of those answers. These answers will be in general terms of what resources you plan to have in your arsenal, under what circumstances will you deploy them, and to what extent you are willing to utilize them.

Decide To Be Ready

Being ready is being fast. At one time, I was a certified chemical weapons (aerosol pepper and teargas) instructor. It amazes me how many civilians carry their pepper spray on their keychain. We all know that attacks often happen right when the victim is getting into their car. The victim is busy, distracted, and easy to shove into the car. So, where is their pepper spray? It's stuck in the door and hanging upside down. If you're not ready to go right now, you're not ready at all.

Decide To Know The Law

Not knowing the law can cause hesitation. That is if you are concerned about the law as you should be. Hesitation is speed lost. While you're trying to decide if it's legal for you to fight back, your attacker, who couldn't care less about laws, will finish you.

I am not an attorney. I have no legal training. I offer you no legal advice. These are just my observations and opinions. As a trained fighter, you will probably be held to a higher standard than someone who is not. To be able to act fast, you must know ahead of time what you can and cannot legally do. Learn as much about self-defense law as possible. When you can use force? How much force you can use? What types of force you can use? The answers vary greatly from one jurisdiction to another. In one place, you may be able to legally stand your ground. In another, you may be required to retreat.

Making It Happen

Whether you want to carry a firearm or not, take a concealed carry course in your jurisdiction. These courses typically go into great depth about use-of-force laws. The course I took covered empty hand situations and less-lethal weapons as well. The instructors are also happy to field questions on this subject. This can be a great resource for beginning to understand use of force laws.

Making It Happen – For This Section

This isn't something that you do just once. Self-defense decisions are a part of your ongoing training. Like the rest of your training, these should be trained to the point of subconscious proficiency with your decisions firmly in your permanent memory ready to be executed by your subconscious mind. The purpose of making these decisions ahead of time is to ensure that, when the time comes for them, your decisions are as sound as possible and as fast as possible.

The result will be that your training can be relied upon and that your conscious mind is freed to process the myriad of unforeseen circumstances that will confront you in a self-defense situation. To be fast during self-defense, you must be as mentally ready as possible.

2. Awareness

Awareness is your key to speed for self-defense situations because you need to know as early as possible that there is a need to defend yourself. That awareness starts long before you have an encounter. That's because the best defense is to never have the encounter at all. The problem is that you don't know when an attack is going to happen.

> *There is only one person who knows*
> *what's going to happen,*
> *when it's going to happen,*
> *and where it's going to happen,*
> *and it is not you.*

Watch people in a shopping center parking lot for a few minutes. I challenge you to find more than one in one hundred that has any clue what is going on around them. They're all sitting ducks. They drive in watching cars and staring down the empty parking spaces. They get out of their car while looking back into the car for their belongings. They walk across the parking lot while staring at their phone or with earbuds in and music blaring. Wolves just love clueless sheep.

So, what's the right way? When you drive into a parking lot, you should notice everything around you. You should be doing this anyway because pedestrians have the right-of-way, and you don't want to run someone down. When you select a parking space, it is in a location where you can see a reasonable perimeter. It's not at the back of the store, away from street lights, and adjoining a thick grove of trees or next to a dumpster. Before you unlock your door, you have a look around. As you exit your car, you don't look back because you collected everything before you ever unlocked the door. In the event that you did forget something, you sit back down, close the door, and lock it. Then, you look around again and exit without looking back. As you walk to the store, you casually look around to the left, right, and behind. If you're self-conscious, pretend that you're looking for someone. Through all of this, you are constantly in the ready to retreat if possible or fight back if necessary. At any point, if it looks like there may be trouble, get away. Now! Not after you ponder about it for a while and worry about what other people think. Get away NOW.

Paranoid?

I stress being aware when I teach self-defense. This sometimes meets resistance.

My female students invariably say to me, "but my friends will all think that I'm paranoid." My response is always the same:

> *"They will call you paranoid until the day that being aware saves you. Then, they'll talk about how smart you are."*

And, who cares if they think that you're paranoid? The alternative is to potentially be violated in unthinkable ways or to die. Yeah, it probably won't happen to you, but that is what nearly every victim thought before it happened to them.

My male self-defense students often take issue with all of this emphasis on awareness and avoidance. They prefer to enumerate the ways they will destroy anybody that dares provoke them. They often take offense with the thought of backing down by avoiding going where they darn well please. To them I say:

> *"Two men in a dark alley are no safer than one woman. So, drop the macho crap."*

When it's time to fight, the sooner that you know an attack is coming the more time you have to respond. Awareness is how you gain time to respond and that is a speed gain. But, there is much more to awareness than fighting. Awareness is your ticket to avoidance and that is the biggest speed gain that you can wish for.

Making It Happen

Awareness starts before you ever leave your house. Know where you're going and what's going to be there. On your way, observe as much as possible at all times. You don't have to do 360's as you walk. Simply scan from left to right. It takes no more than a couple of seconds. If you see something that troubles you, back off. Don't take chances. A little delay is worth it.

3. When It's Time To Fight

You've done everything that you can to avoid threatening situations. You've avoided dangerous places. You've tried to walk away. You've complied with the bad person's demands, and you've been non-confrontational. You've done all that you can do to avoid harming anyone. And still, violence has been thrust upon you.

I am not suggesting that you do anything that puts you in greater danger. Everything that I just listed is meant to get you out of harm's way, not to get you in deeper. Often absolutely none of that will work and you are immediately forced to fight back. In that case, fight to win.

This is when your training should kick in. All of that work that you've done to fill your permanent memory and subconscious mind with effective technique and good decisions is your best hope. That training is what will make you fast and effective. The decisions you made before this ever happened have freed your conscious mind so it can process at peak efficiency dealing with the massive decision-making the situation will demand. Make no mistake, your conscious mind will be hard at work because it is impossible to anticipate everything that will happen in a self-defense situation. That is why you have moved as much as possible to your permanent memory and subconscious mind. You need all of the conscious thinking capacity possible to ensure that you make safe, effective, and legal decisions.

Speed for Self-Defense

Be Efficient

Most of what is taught as self-defense is extraordinarily inefficient and slow. If your self-defense techniques require multiple moves, extreme accuracy, spins, or exaggerated body positions, abandon them now. It is imperative that self-defense techniques exact as much damage as possible as quickly and efficiently as possible.

When It's Time, It's Time

There's an old sci-fi movie entitled *"The Last Star Fighter."* In the movie, space aliens were in a search for new fighter pilots to help defend their world. They placed an arcade-style video game on earth as a clandestine way to test earthlings in a search for the job. Score big on the video game and you end up fighting actual space battles. A reluctant teenage guy from the middle of nowhere gets to make the trip. In his fighter craft, there was a red button that his instructor warned him to never press. It turns out to be the fighter pilot's last hope in the face of overwhelming odds. Desperate and against overwhelming odds is right where he eventually finds himself, so we get to see what the red button is all about. The button gets pressed, and the tiny fighter craft begins to spin and fire everything that it has in all directions rapid fire, with speed and fury. It looked like a spinning fireworks display. When it had expended everything it had, there wasn't a single enemy craft left.

What's the point? You're only fighting because you have absolutely no other choice. In that case, in my opinion, it's time to expend everything that you are. This also doesn't mean indiscriminately thrashing about. It means systematically, efficiently, and accurately giving everything that you've got to effect a decisive victory in a fight that has been forced upon you.

There have been many cases in which sport martial artists have been defeated in the street because they fought as if there were rules and limits. Self-defense requires everything you've got. It's all business, and you've got to be all in. Turn off emotion, and get the job done. Remember though, you are defending, not punishing. If you exceed your assailant's aggression, it is possible that you will become the aggressor in the eyes of the law.

Surprise

Nothing is faster than a surprise attack. Surprise attacks can be devastating as well. However, there are problems with surprise attacks for self-defense. Usually, it is the victim that is surprised. There are many ways for the victim to take advantage of the element of surprise though. All of them carry serious risks, but you wouldn't be fighting if you had any other choice, right?

The Risks

I can't discuss something as risky as surprise attacks without addressing the risk involved. The biggest risks in a surprise attack, by you as a victim, are the same as any time that you fight back. You may lose and you may elevate the threat. Surprise attacks add the risk of potentially finding yourself on the wrong side of the law. For the victim to take advantage of the element of surprise, there must be a break in the action. Initiating an attack during that break can cause you to be considered the aggressor because your attacker may be considered to have disengaged. When being held captive, when you are under threat of a weapon, or when you are faking defeat, but your attacker is still advancing, are times that you might be able to legally use a surprise attack. Unfortunately, you won't know until after it is all over. That's why you must know as much about the laws governing self-defense as possible. See "Know The Law" in the "Decisions" section above.

Making It Happen

Using the element of surprise fits right in with avoidance because while you are trying to avoid a fight you are also constantly looking for an opening to exploit.

Faking Compliance - I've told my kids since they were old enough to understand me that I will work up a tear if I can get an assailant to drop his hands. That's right. The black belt is going to appear as scared as possible. I'm going to be as non-confrontational as I can be. I'm going to give the bad guy what he wants. I'm going to do everything that I can to convince my assailant that I'm not going to fight back and if he will leave me alone I won't. The entire time though, I'm going to be looking for an opening in the event that I need it. And, if I have no other choice, I am going to drive through that opening with everything that I am, and I'm not going to stop until the threat is neutralized.

When do I want my assailant to know that I'm going to fight back? Shortly after impact.

Now, I could have jumped into a fighting stance and maybe even threw in a nice loud kiai. First, that is probably going to escalate the situation. Second, it would take away any element of surprise that I may have had. Third, it's just stupid.

Choreography And Scripting Are Death To Speed

For crying out loud, abandon choreography and scripting. Martial art instructors have had a tremendously long love affair with choreographed and scripted self-defense training. Does anyone actually think that any of that stuff is going to work in the street? The techniques taught in this way are typically exaggerated and require a high level of precision. They are typically extraordinarily slow, not to mention terribly ineffective. They invariably require a cooperative assailant.

Learn fast, efficient, and effective techniques. Then, gear up heavily and make your self-defense practice as unpredictable and realistic as you can safely make it. Incorporate simple and devastatingly effective techniques that attack vulnerable areas as efficiently as possible. All of that facilitates speed. Remember, effective completion is your goal.

Groin Strikes May Be A Waste Of Time

And therefore, a waste of speed. Men are conditioned from a very early age to instinctively protect the groin area. For that reason, they can do so extremely fast. Protection is reflex rather than response (which means that the nervous system bypasses the brain). It doesn't get any faster than reflex. If you are going to attack the groin, ensure that you have a very clear opening with a very high probability of success, or you're wasting time and effort. Given that you must be very close for a groin attack, you are also going to leave yourself vulnerable should the attack fail. If attacking with your hands, your guard will be down as well during the attack so attack fast, accurately, and rechamber immediately.

Sloppy Is Fast

Huh? Not sloppy like you're thinking. By sloppy, I mean techniques that don't attempt to pinpoint vulnerable targets. Do you really think you can eye jab a crazed attacker while you are scared for your life and you're both moving erratically? I doubt it.

For self-defense, I prefer what I call "sloppy" techniques. Sloppy techniques are as wide as possible and have multiple chances for success. They are easy to execute when compared to techniques that require precision. Their primary speed factor is that they are more assured of reaching effective completion, which is always your ultimate goal. They are also fast because they are easy to execute.

Making It Happen

These are just a couple of examples. The idea is to use a wide weapon across multiple vulnerable targets that uses a motion that is easy to execute.

- **Head** – Use a clawing-type hand position like you are going to rake your fingernails across something. Your hand will be open with full exposure of your palm. In a sweeping motion, strike the side of the head at a slight downward angle continuing across the face. Your first target is the palm of the hand to the ear. If you are slightly off target, that motion can impact the temple with the palm heel. If those miss, you can claw the eyes. If that misses, your nails can scratch the face deeply. Then hopefully, you will snag the lower lip and tear it. You can easily lose a fingernail or two, or even dislocate or break a finger in the process, but you will inflict a lot of damage along the way. That's worth it.

- **Leg** – This attack uses a short forward stepping motion. As you step, lift your foot high enough to impact the knee. Your foot should be slightly turned inward for a knife-edge impact. This provides a wide weapon. As you step forward, put your foot down hard in a stomping motion that has a slight forward angle. Your first target is the top of the kneecap. If that misses, you can scrape down the shin. If that misses, hopefully you will deliver a solid stomp to the foot. If all of that misses, you will land in a stable position having only taken a step forward. That forward motion will be great for delivering an elbow or forearm impact to the throat or solar plexus.

Stay As Relaxed As Possible

You know what it feels like to nearly fall backward in a chair? Your heart pounds and your stomach fills with a blast of acid. You spend the next few minutes coming down from the adrenalin rush. Well, your first self-defense encounter will feel like a nuclear version of that.

The adrenalin rush alone can be paralyzing. Your training will mitigate some of the effects because, if nothing else, it won't be the first time that someone has taken a swing at you, even if it was expected in training. The more realistic your training, the more relaxed you can be when it becomes real. It should be real enough to get a little scary. Keep it safe but with enough pressure to take you well out of your comfort zone. That's because fear is debilitating. It's something that you must overcome. Gear up heavily and work with someone you can't beat. Let them scare you. Survive and then do it again.

To be fast, to make use of your training, and to make good conscious decisions, you must be as relaxed as possible. The decisions you made in the first section of this chapter will help tremendously. There are few things that will calm you more than knowing ahead of time how you will handle a situation. Even more important though is to make a decision that wasn't mentioned in that section. Decide to be relaxed. Yup, simple as that. I didn't say that it's easy; I said that it's simple. You have more control over yourself than you probably currently exert. Decide to stay calm because being nervous can cause you to fail when you otherwise would have succeeded. Be scared later, be worried later, be angry later. Right now, it's all business. Focus only on success. That may be avoidance, flight, compliance, or fighting back. Regardless, stay calm and on task. Whether you think so or not, you can do that. See "Is There A Nurse In The House?" (page 155).

Sharing Your Weapon With Your Attacker

Never give away a speed advantage. Any weapon that is not in use, and is the same distance from you as it is from your opponent, is a shared weapon (hands, feet, and anything else you use to fight with is a weapon). Your attacker can get to it just as quickly as you can put it into use. It's just a matter of who moves first. You may be faster, but you're defending. That means you most likely aren't going to be moving first.

If you put a knife to my throat and hold it there to threaten me, I will easily take it from you before you can even begin to move it. That's because it is so close that you can't perceive and respond to my motion before my defensive movement is over. An extended arm is a gift to a grappler or even an untrained opponent because it can easily be grabbed before you can retract it. If you're holding a weapon, it may end up in the hands of your opponent. Keep your weapons closer to you than they are to your opponent lest they end up being used against you. Only move a weapon close to your opponent when it is on its way to its target.

Bibliography

Conrad, B., Benecke, R., & Goehmann, M. (1983). Premovement silent period in fast movement initiation. *Experimental Brain Research, 51*, 310-313.

Gillen, J.B., Martin, B.J., MacInnis, M.J., Shelly, L.E., Tamopolsky, M.A. & Gibala, M.J. (2016). Twelve weeks of sprint interval training improves indices of cardiometabolic health similar to traditional endurance training despite a five-fold lower exercise volume and time commitment. *PLOS ONE, 11*(4). Retrieved October 20, 2016, from http://doi.org/10.1371/journal.pone.0154075

Heinzel, A., Ross, H-G., & Cleveland, S. (2008). Antagonist muscle activation preceding rapid flexion movements of the elbow joint in human subjects. *Neuroscience Letters, 434,* 206-211.

Hummelscheim, H., & Hefter, H. (1991). A premovement silent period does not occur prior to rapid changes of velocity during human limb movements. *Neuroscience Letters, 124,* 52-56.

Kottke, F.J. (1980). From reflex to skill: the training of coordination. *Arch Phys Med Rehabil, 61,* 551-561.

Mortimer, J.A., Eisenberg, P., & Palmer, S.S. (1987). Premovement silence in agonist muscles preceding maximum efforts. *Experimental Neurology, 98,* 542-554.

Walter, C.B. (1988). The influence of agonist premotor silence and the stretch-shortening cycle on contractile rate in active skeletal muscles. *European Journal of Applied Physiology, 57,* 577-582.

About the Author

David Howell brings a unique combination of skills to the study of speed. His martial art studies began in 1980. He has trained in many varied styles and had a very successful tournament career to which he credits his speed. He has also studied the mind, learning ability, and intelligence for over 36 years. He teaches accelerated learning and high-level cognitive skills. Howell takes a very analytical approach to the study of speed. Conversely, he takes a plain-spoken, no-nonsense approach to teaching that is focused on maximum results.

www.TheBookofSpeed.com

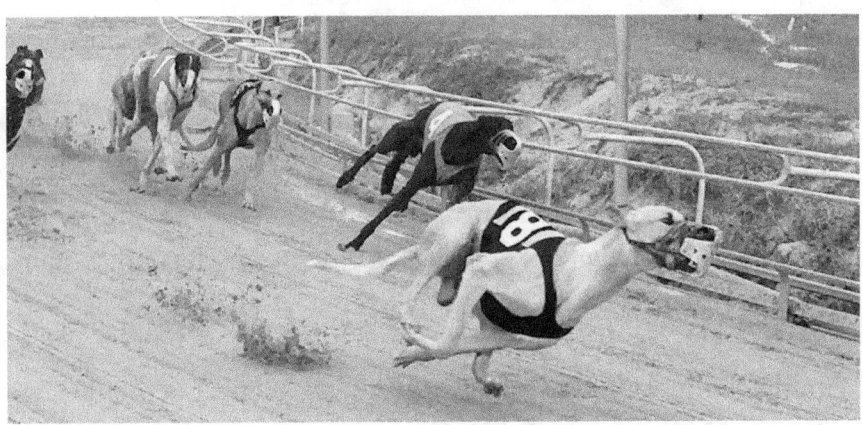

Photo by Kathi Lacasse

Even His Dogs Are Fast

Howell and his family have adopted several retired racing greyhounds. They're the second fastest land animal on the planet, and they love to run, but they're just as happy lounging on your sofa. They make great pets, and they'll help keep you fast.

Make a fast friend. Adopt a greyhound.
Adopt-A-Greyhound.org

www.ingramcontent.com/pod-product-compliance
Lightning Source LLC
LaVergne TN
LVHW051548070426
835507LV00021B/2466